Staying

Alive

Healing from Heart Disease

A Survivor's Story

SHERRY SHRALLOW

WHAT PEOPLE ARE SAYING ABOUT *STAYING ALIVE*

Sherry Shrallow has been an inspiration to me since my husband and I attended her adult education class on heart healthy nutrition and cooking. I had been interested in preparing meals that support heart health but struggled to find resources. Sherry provided the tools for healthy eating and meal preparation; simple tasty recipes, cooking demonstrations, and motivating information from her extensive studies in the area of nutritional support for optimal cardiovascular health. She generously shares her personal experiences that fueled her passion for heart health and has been a powerful support in helping others to transform their health. She has the gift of making complex medical information accessible and relevant. She has also helped me (a non-cook) build a repertoire of quick, tasty, healthy meals in a wide variety of cuisines. My lipid panels show her influence! I am so grateful that I have had the opportunity of changing my health through Sherry's help. I wish everyone could have this experience!

Susan Nash
Libertyville, Illinois

Staying Alive is the real life story of Sherry Shrallow, a vibrant 56 year-old psychotherapist who came face to face with early mortality and in an unlikely process discovered that she could reverse the disease that almost claimed her life. Having worked with Sherry in our psychotherapy practice, I would never have thought that that this could happen to her. She was a physically fit woman who exercised regularly and who ate what she thought was a healthy Mediterranean diet. Her story will show you how determined she became to take care of her own health by following a whole foods, oil-free plant-based diet based on the science she learned about from Dr. Caldwell Esselstyn, Jr. in his book *Prevent and Reverse Heart Disease*. Sherry has been a relentless advocate on the subject of plant-based nutrition, combatting misinformation presented to the public as she teaches classes on heart disease prevention and reversal and engages students in cooking classes in her own home. Accurate scientific information is powerful when shared. If it's up to Sherry, *Staying Alive* will never be a secret.

Dawn Nelson LCSW
Houston, Texas

Until I met Sherry Shrallow, I always believed I led a healthy lifestyle. A competitive runner for 40+ years, I blamed my achy, inflamed joints, frequent headaches, sinus infections, and increasingly high blood pressure on aging, allergies, and over-training. After all, didn't my diet include generous helpings of lean meat, dairy, and olive oil? (Full disclosure: a goodly amount of sugar too.) Through her own inspiring story of survival and transformation, Sherry offers a sensible, non-judgmental alternative to the medications doctors are so quick to prescribe and the misinformation spewed by Big Food. After watching *Forks Over Knives* and reading *The China Study*, I transitioned to a mostly oil-free whole foods plant-based diet with Sherry's guidance and encouragement. The results were swift and impressive. In a matter of months, all of my symptoms were greatly reduced or disappeared entirely! As I continue on this journey, I'm grateful for experts like Sherry who generously share their knowledge, passion, and empathy as they challenge the entrenched status quo. She is among the world's most respected voices spearheading a grassroots movement that is changing lives for the better, one healthy eater at a time.

John Gagliardi
Lake Zurich, Illinois

DEDICATION

This book is dedicated to my soulmate and loving husband, Dale, to my children, Michael, Joel and Allison, to my daughter-in-law Heather, to my son-in-law Tim, and to the two new loves of my life, my grandchildren, Ethan and Aubrey.

Writing a book was certainly a new undertaking for me. I want to thank two very special people who assisted me on my journey. Joan Rosemarin—dear friend, former neighbor and member of my mah jongg group—thank you so much for sitting with me for hours on end, helping me to get my book off the ground. The writing skills that Joan, a recently retired English teacher, brought to bear proved invaluable to me. And Dale, my always supportive husband, I thank you for going over each and every line in this book with me numerous times until we got it just right. Your editing skills are incredible, and I couldn't have done this without you.

I also dedicate this book to the memory of every person who has lost his or her life prematurely to heart disease. May this book empower those suffering with this disease to survive and thrive simply by changing what they eat for breakfast, lunch and dinner, and may it also inspire those without heart disease to be proactive in taking steps to ensure they never develop it.

Table of Contents

INTRODUCTION

If you want to travel fast, go alone.
If you want to travel far, go together.
African proverb

Within the pages of this heartfelt book, Sherry will be your companion as you take a journey that tells the story of her personal health crisis, healing, transformation and resilience. In the most human way it will connect your heart with hers and will remind you that even under the most difficult of circumstances there is the chance to appreciate the precious nature of life, gain insight and cultivate compassion. You will be inspired by her ability to transform her personal suffering into wisdom and action that is helping countless people improve the health of their bodies, minds and spirits and healing this beautiful home we call Mother Earth. The information and recipes will inspire you to nourish your life.

Sherry and I first became acquainted in a yoga class I was teaching. She was a friendly and familiar student who attended regularly but I did not know her personally. Even so, I was sorry to see her go when she informed me that her husband's work was taking them from the suburbs of Chicago to Houston. I remember that shortly after she moved there was a severe hurricane in Houston, and I wished for her safety. She was safe although shaken from that storm but a different sort of hurricane was about to take her through an unexpected health event that nearly ended her life.

Sherry's journey from surviving to thriving was challenging and sometimes frustrating as she navigated through both the good and bad of the modern American health care system. While in recovery she was awakened to the science and practices linking diet and disease, somewhat out of the mainstream American dietary philosophies, which guided her toward being an active participant in her return to vibrant health. Motivated to change her diet, she set upon a path that wasn't easy. It required patience, time, study, trial and error and personal discipline. Sometimes it meant enduring the criticisms of doctors and friends who judged her choices as too extreme. It required that she trust that soft and true voice of inner wisdom and have faith that her actions were steady and sound.

When Sherry returned to Chicago and came back to my yoga class I was delighted. As we reconnected following that first class, she told me her story openly and with a sense of palpable peace and purpose. I have witnessed her dedication to learning about the science and lifestyle of eating a whole foods plant-based diet. She *lives* this practice and opens her heart and home to help and support others in this lifestyle choice and to do her part in helping to heal Mother Earth and preserve her bounty for future generations. Her philosophy is not about deprivation—it is about abundance.

Sherry is a sought-after therapist and dedicates herself professionally to helping people understand the nature of the mind, patterns and behaviors so that they can live happier, kinder and more fulfilled lives. Most importantly, Sherry models the way to live with vibrant health, purpose and love. She takes time to be in nature, to move her body, to practice yoga, qi gong and meditation daily. She is gentle with herself, her family and friends while remaining steady and strong on the path of peace and healing.

May Sherry's story inspire and inform you to live your life in the most authentic way. If you need to make some changes, may this be the spark that ignites the fire within to embark upon a new journey of healing, discovery and transformation. If you are well upon this path, may her story be your companion so that you can travel further than you even imagined, with Sherry by your side. Along with her, may you always know the precious nature of your life. May the thoughts and words she shares bring you insight, peace and happiness.

Ceily Levy
Taos, New Mexico
July 2017

1

The Day That Changed My Life

November 16, 2010, was a gorgeous day in Houston, Texas. I loved this time of year when I could go outside with only a light jacket or sweater and enjoy the warmth. It had been a typical workday for me. Having just finished seeing my last psychotherapy client for the day, I planned to go home to rest for a few hours before facilitating an executive women's support group at a local restaurant that evening.

Before leaving the office, I decided to return a phone call to the father of one of my adolescent clients. Without warning, a feeling of nausea overtook me during our conversation. At the same time, I broke out in a cold sweat from head to toe and felt light-headed. Having just returned from lunch, I wondered if something I had eaten wasn't sitting well in my stomach. I could hardly concentrate on what the father was saying to me on the phone, and all I knew was that I had to end the call quickly. So I said to him "I'm sorry but I have to go. I have a client waiting to see me." I hung up abruptly without even waiting for him to say goodbye. Sitting on my sofa, I felt myself slipping into darkness, ultimately losing consciousness.

When I came to, I immediately thought, "I'm having a heart attack!" Knowing that time was of the essence, I realized I had to get medical help immediately. Thank goodness, I had taken time to call that father back before leaving my office. Otherwise I could have been driving home when I lost consciousness, possibly running off the road, killing myself or hurting someone in my path. It was then that I managed to pick up my cell phone and call my husband, Dale, and uttered the words, "Honey I'm sick. I think I'm having a heart attack. Call 911."

For privacy reasons, my office door was always locked when I was seeing patients. Somehow, I knew that I had to get myself to that door to unlock it so that the paramedics could get to me. There was no time to waste! I have no idea how I found the strength to crawl across the room to unlock it. Once open, I collapsed onto the floor. Crying out "Help!" as loudly as I could. I kept hoping that the therapist in the next office would hear me, but, unfortunately, he never did. I remember saying to myself, "This is it, I'm going to die." Finally, a man sitting in the waiting room heard me yelling and ran over to my office. Seeing me sprawled out on the floor, he immediately alerted the other therapist. At the same time, to my great relief, the paramedics arrived, having received my husband's call. All of this took no more than 15 minutes.

Wasting no time, the first responders asked me a few questions, checked my vital signs, and gave me an aspirin. My worst fears were confirmed when the paramedic said to me, "This might be a heart attack." They quickly put me on a gurney to make the trip down four floors to the awaiting ambulance. Unfortunately, the elevator in my building was too narrow to accommodate the gurney in the supine position, so they had to sit me up for the ride down. My head was spinning from being upright, but they had no choice if they wanted to get me out of there. I was conscious at that time and acutely aware of my life-threatening situation. Reading the paramedics report years later, I discovered that I had said to them, "I feel doom coming upon me."

Now outside, I found Dale, having raced from his office to be by my side, waiting for me by the ambulance. Consistent with what the paramedics had told me, I overheard one of them telling him he thought I was having a heart attack. They got me into the ambulance and within five minutes we arrived at the nearest hospital. Dazed, I kept asking myself, "Is this really happening?"

Once in the emergency room, with Dale by my side, I turned to him and said "Honey, please call Liz and tell her I probably won't be able to make it to the group tonight." How silly of me, worrying about work during a heart attack. But that's me, Miss-Responsible-All-The-Way. As the cardiologist rushed into the room, I looked him in the eye and said, "Please don't let me die." He met my gaze with equal intensity and promised "I won't."

Unfortunately, his promise was almost broken. When under sedation in the procedure room the cardiologist inserted a catheter into my 99% blocked right coronary artery. Suddenly I vomited. The sudden movement caused the catheter to shift, dissecting my aorta. This was a major complication. Without immediate bypass surgery and repair of my torn aorta, death was now a certainty. On his way into the operating room, the chief surgeon stopped and told Dale, "You'd better call your family and get them here as fast as you can. I don't think your wife's going to make it. I give her at best a 20% chance of surviving." My poor husband. He must have been reeling from such a dire forecast. How was he going to tell our children that their mother would likely die?

The only thing I remember while in that operating suite was being shocked by the defibrillator on one of the three occasions when my heart stopped beating that day and I came to for a moment, shouting, "Ouch...That hurts!" It was hard to believe this was happening to me. I was only 56 years old, the same age as my grandfather when he died suddenly from a heart attack. Was history going to repeat itself?

2

Signs and Symptoms

Thankfully I survived.

What was so baffling to me and to everyone I knew was that, by all appearances, I had been a very healthy woman prior to this event. I ate well, consuming a Mediterranean-style diet, was of normal weight, and exercised almost every day doing either aerobics, swimming, walking, running, yoga, cross country skiing or weight training. It didn't make sense that I would have heart disease in the prime of my life. But I did. How could this happen? After all, I had no outward symptoms of heart disease...or did I?

Consider this: Four years earlier, on a flight back from Israel, scrunched into my economy seat, I decided to take the sleeping pill Ambien to sleep through the night flight. Big mistake. When I arrived home in Chicago, I noticed I was limping on my left leg when walking towards the baggage claim area. The limp was soon accompanied by a shooting pain.

The next day, when the pain continued, I told a friend of mine about it. She sounded very concerned and told me to get myself to my doctor immediately, which I did. It turned out that I had a blood clot in my leg. My doctor thought it was because I hadn't gotten up to move around during the ten-hour flight home. Sitting that long can cause clotting to occur in the legs. I was put on Warfarin for 6 months, after which my physician told me that the clot had dissolved. I thought all was well.

Looking back, the blood clot in my leg may have been a sign about the condition of my vascular system, but there were other signs as well.

Four months before my heart attack my sister and I enjoyed a week-long vacation at The Chautauqua Institute in New York. I had been jogging regularly by then, and on one of my daily runs I remember feeling unusually tired. Fighting that fatigue, I somehow managed to finish the run. I attributed the tiredness that I felt to the hills that dotted the course. Nevertheless, afterwards, I just didn't feel well and felt sapped of all my energy, but I couldn't pinpoint any specific cause.

My sister and I had always loved playing tennis together. During one of our matches that week in New York, I again experienced an overwhelming fatigue. It was a doubles match, and we were playing against two great competitors. Always wanting to win, I was racing around that court like a mad woman, trying to get to every ball so that I could send it sailing back over that net. We ended up losing the match but did not go down without a fight. I once again chalked the fatigue up to getting older, not having played tennis for many years, and facing two ferocious players.

Several months passed without any further warnings. Then, in October of 2010, my husband and I were at our friend's son's wedding in Baltimore. This was about three weeks before I had my heart attack. For those of you who may not be familiar with downtown Baltimore, there is a very lovely area called the Inner Harbor, where Dale and I stayed. We had decided to go for our respective runs before the evening festivities. I remember feeling really, really tired once again when I started to run and after 10 minutes or so, I had to walk the rest of the way. Back at the hotel, I lay down to rest, feeling like I had just been hit by a Mack truck. In no way did I think that this had anything to do with the exhaustion I had experienced in New York several months earlier.

At the wedding that evening I felt fine enough, dancing the whole night long. However, the next morning, at a brunch for the wedding guests, I felt awful. My head hurt, I was sneezing, had a runny nose, and could barely keep my eyes open. At the airport later that day, all I could do was sit and try to sleep in my chair at our gate while waiting to board our plane. That was not like me. I usually walk up and down the concourse to pass the time before flying, getting some exercise in before having to sit still for the next several hours.

After we arrived home later that afternoon, I shopped for groceries for the coming week, since we hardly had any food in the house. Pushing that grocery cart through the aisles felt as if I was pushing it through wet cement. I was moving in slow motion. All I wanted to do was to get out of there, get home, get in my pajamas, and go to sleep. "This is some cold I've got," I kept telling myself. But sure enough, the virus left me, and within a few days I started feeling better. I went back to running on the treadmill in our condo's exercise room and all seemed fine.

Meanwhile, I was under tremendous work pressure to create a presentation for the Executive Women's Committee of The Greater Houston Partnership. At the same time, I was working full time in my psychotherapy practice. I felt under the gun trying to juggle all aspects of my work and personal life. Once again, I attributed my exhaustion to trying to do too much at one time, and I shrugged it off.

After my near-death experience, I wanted to fully understand the signs and symptoms of a heart attack. Checking out the American Heart Association's website[1] here's what I learned.

According to the American Heart Association, a person having a heart attack may experience discomfort in the center of the chest that lasts more than a few minutes or that goes away and comes back. It can feel like uncomfortable pressure, squeezing, fullness or pain. Pain can also be felt in one or both arms, the back, neck, jaw or stomach. Shortness of breath, with or without chest discomfort, can also signal a heart attack. These are not the only symptoms, however, and, in fact, I experienced none of them. Rather, my heart attack was accompanied by perhaps lesser known factors—a cold sweat, nausea, lightheadedness and fainting. Lucky for me, I had known about these less obvious symptoms and had acted upon them. For women who don't, the consequences can be deadly. Further, it is not uncommon for women who do report these symptoms to their doctors to be misdiagnosed. The lesson here is to listen to your body—if something feels off, check it out immediately. Don't assume it's nothing. Be respectfully assertive with your doctor. If you have any of these sudden symptoms wherever you are, do not hesitate to call 911. It's better to be safe than sorry. Thank goodness I didn't hesitate and did just that. Remember, heart disease can take your life in a second, even before you know what hit you. There are no do-overs. Heart disease is the number one killer of men and women in the United States.

November 16, 2010, the day of my heart attack, bypass surgery and near-death experience, set in motion a whole new life for me.

3

The Hospital

My new life began in the Intensive Care Unit. "Normal" as I had known it had just flown out the window and had no intention of returning any time soon. My new normal left me feeling weak, unable to care for myself, and dependent upon others. It appeared I had a long road ahead of me.

In critical condition post-surgery, I remained in the Surgical Intensive Care Unit for seven days. My chest was left open because I required a Right Ventricle Assist Device (RVAD) to keep me alive until my heart was strong enough to work on its own again. Much to the surprise of my surgeon, who expected me to be on the machine for at least five days, I was taken off the device in only two days. He was amazed that my heart had recovered enough in that short period of time, but he was more than happy to remove the RVAD and close my chest. Perhaps it had been how fit I was from all of my regular exercising prior to my heart attack that helped me get off that machine ahead of schedule.

Dale later told me that there was a representative from the RVAD company regularly standing at the foot of my bed to ensure it functioned properly. There was no room for error. If it somehow malfunctioned, I would die. So focused on the machine's workings, that representative never looked at Dale nor said a word to him. I had at least eight tubes inserted into different parts of my chest and neck area. I was on a ventilator, kept in a sedated state, with no memory of anything that was going on around me. I was like a Sleeping Beauty, but much less attractive, with a body that had filled with fluid that made me look like an overinflated balloon. It is still hard for my family to talk to me about how scary I looked, unrecognizable from the person they knew.

My surgeon told Dale, "Your wife's going to need a pacemaker." Once again, I proved him incorrect. My heart fully recovered, and a pacemaker was never needed. I guess he didn't know me. I am a tough cookie.

Many people have asked me, "What do you remember about your time in the ICU?" I tell them, "Nothing, except for one thing." It was my daughter Allison, who had flown in from San Francisco, who was able to grab my attention. You see, Allison has a very strong personality. If she wants you to hear her, she will make that happen. I remember her saying in a loud, clear voice, "Mom, I love you. Squeeze my hand if you can hear me." I couldn't speak because of the breathing tube that was down my throat, but I clearly heard her command. All I could do was to raise one hand and, using my own version of sign language, tell her, "I (pointing at myself) love (pointing at my heart) you" (pointing in her direction).

My next stop after the ICU was to a medical surgical floor in the hospital, where I stayed for another week. My memories from that time are virtually nonexistent. Who took care of me? How did I eat? Who were my doctors? Nothing. Thinking back, I am glad I have so few recollections from my hospital stay. Amnesia can be a blessing, and for me it was. It is fascinating how the mind protects us from trauma by blocking out those memories, as my situation was way too much for my psyche to absorb and process during that time.

When I was able to speak again, I asked Dale, "What happened to me?" He hesitated and said, "Do you really want to know right now?" I said, "Yes, I do." Knowing me as well as he did, he knew he couldn't dodge the bullet any longer, so he told me. I was stunned. With tears running down my cheeks I cried out, "How could this have happened?" It was at that moment, lying in my hospital bed, that I realized I had to find the answer and try to make sure this never happened to me again.

Dale must have been terrified during those first few weeks. We had been in Houston for only two years and were far from family and friends who lived in other parts of the country. The day of my heart attack, Dale called Liz, the woman who had hired me to coach the Executive Women's group, to tell her what had happened. She came immediately to the hospital and stayed right by his side in the surgical waiting room all night long. Her presence and support helped Dale get through that very long night. When I was finally in the ICU, Dale made his way home, trying to get some sleep with our two cats snuggled up against him, frightened and worried and asking himself, "Is this the day Sherry is going to die?"

One of the hardest things he had to do was to tell family and friends what had happened to me. In order to not be inundated with calls and emails, he kept his call list short, and asked one friend to regularly update everyone else we knew about my condition. Dale was in no shape to be on the phone as his focus was on being with me in the hospital. From what I learned later, everyone was shocked beyond belief. "If it happened to Sherry, could this happen to me?" One friend was so worried about her own heart that she made an appointment with a cardiologist to discuss some of her own unsettling cardiac symptoms as soon as she got the news about me.

Dale spent every day with me in the hospital, sitting quietly by my bedside, making sure I was being well taken care of. We were visited by two local rabbis and a cantor who prayed for my recovery on several occasions. He was also comforted by a temple congregant whom he had never met but who became aware of what had happened to me. Those visits proved to be very comforting to Dale. I, of course, have no memory of those visits or any others. Our Houston friends came by the hospital to sit with and comfort Dale. Everyone was praying for us, including my brother and sister who flew in.

Dale and I were a close couple who discussed everything, but during that time, when I was out of it, he no longer had that connection with me. All he could do was be present at my bedside, hold my hand, and hope for the best. As one of my surgeons wrote in my medical chart, my situation was dire.

There was one comical moment that deserves telling, although it wasn't so funny at the time to our son Michael. Dale, Michael and our daughter Allison had just arrived home from a long day at the hospital when Dale told them he'd be back in a minute. He went down to the lobby of our building to pick up our mail, and when he returned he found our son Michael screaming hysterically at his sister. "What in the world is going on here" asked a confused Dale. Allison had recently taken the California Bar exam and was anxiously awaiting her results. When she checked her score online she ran into the living room screaming at the top of her lungs, "I passed! I passed!" Michael ran out of his bedroom shouting at his sister "What do you mean she passed?" He thought she was telling him that I had just passed in the hospital. Talk about a misunderstanding, but at least someone had some good news to tell that terrible day.

After two long weeks in the hospital, it was finally time for me to leave. I was being moved to a rehabilitation center to continue my recovery. No homecoming for me just yet.

4

Off to the Rehabilitation Center

The hospital had been my safe haven for the past two weeks and leaving left me with feelings of tremendous apprehension. Although I was no longer in critical condition, I was in no condition to go home.

So, on a crisp evening in early December, I was wheeled down to the hospital's lobby and got into our car for Dale to drive the short distance to the rehabilitation center (RC). Upon arrival, we were greeted by a nurse who accompanied us to my room on the third floor. The nurse checked my vital signs, asked me a lot of questions and then left as I settled into my new bed. When it was time for Dale to leave that evening, I remember feeling terribly sad, knowing that I could not go home with him. I was still so weak, unable to tend to my basic needs, and dependent on strangers to take care of me. Tears welled up in my eyes as I kissed Dale goodbye that night. Lying slightly upright in my hospital bed, I tried to sleep, but found it difficult as I kept replaying over and over in my mind all that had happened to me.

The next morning, I was greeted by one of the nurse's aides, who helped get me out of bed, dressed, and into a wheelchair. She was very kind and understanding. My fears were beginning to subside a bit in this new, strange place after this one encounter with this lovely, empathic nurse's aide. She wheeled me down to the dining room and placed me at one of the long rectangular tables, lined with elderly people on each side, each quietly eating their breakfast. I was presented with a tray of eggs, juice, coffee and toast, but I had no appetite. Even looking at that food made me feel nauseous. All I felt like doing was putting my head down on that table and sobbing.

My tablemates were mostly there to recover from falls or strokes. A woman sitting across from me at breakfast that first day was recovering from a fall, but she also had severe dementia. She kept repeating the same things over and over again to me. I was only 56 years old and felt so out of place. How did I end up here? It just seemed impossible that this was what my life was now about. Now don't get me wrong, I love elderly people. I had worked with them for years as a professional social worker, but I was not prepared to be part of this rehab community in my mid-fifties.

What really struck me as odd about my first meal were the eggs they had put on my plate. I'd just had a heart attack and knew enough to question the rationale behind serving me a food that was laden with cholesterol—a well-known contributor to heart disease. Eggs actually have the most cholesterol of any food, composed of 272MG/100 Cal as compared with beef, which has 33MG/100 Cal.[2] Questioning the dietician in charge of my case about the wisdom of serving a heart attack survivor eggs for breakfast, I was told she was most concerned about my sodium intake and not the eggs. Even in my weakened and depressed state, I knew intuitively that she should have been equally concerned about my cholesterol intake.

Lunch and dinner were much the same when it came to animal cholesterol. Both meals had either chicken or beef as the main course, neither of which I could stomach. For some reason, animal protein became a big concern for those taking care of me, and they wanted me to eat as much of it as possible. Having read my medical records from my hospital stay, the nutritionist there even noted in my chart that she was concerned I was not getting enough animal protein and was thrilled to report that I ate the meat in my sandwich one day! So, I asked the dietician at the RC about getting some fish instead and she graciously accommodated my request, but it was so unappealing to me once it arrived on my plate that it was left uneaten, along with everything else they served me. By the time I left the RC, I weighed 114 pounds, down 16 pounds from where I had started.

Participating in physical and occupational therapy became part of my daily routine. I could barely walk from my bed to the bathroom in my room and needed help getting dressed and bathed, making me wonder if I would ever regain my former strength. My walker became my main mode of transportation, getting me from point A to point B, no matter how short a distance I had to travel. Trying to walk from my room to the dining room, which was just down the hallway, seemed like a cross country trek! Even short distances left me exhausted and in need of an immediate nap.

My physical therapist was a no-nonsense kind of gal. She had me pedaling a bike twice a day along with a host of other strengthening exercises. To say I was whipped after each session would be quite an understatement. There were many days when I would have been happy to have been left alone in my bed, but that was not to be. She would come to my room if I wasn't on that bike at the designated time and kindly yet firmly get me up and into that physical therapy room. On one day, she had in mind that I would walk up four steps. Looking at her as though she was crazy, I said, "You've got to be kidding!" Well, she wasn't. She made me do it, and when I got to the top, panting and sweating, I felt like I had climbed Mount Everest! That's the kind of physical therapist she was, moving me forward in my recovery even when I resisted.

My occupational therapist was charged with teaching me how to safely dress, shower myself and perform the normal activities of daily living. At first, I couldn't even put on a pair of slippers without assistance. Just getting out of my nightgown took so much effort that I had to rest before attempting to put on my workout clothes for the day. The open-heart surgery had left me with a frozen shoulder, a condition where moving the arm in an upright position was nearly impossible and very painful. Try taking off a shirt or putting on a pair of pants when your arm aches and will not cooperate—not an easy feat.

My surgery left me with wounds up and down my chest and neck area that needed daily cleaning. One was particularly large, located in the middle of my chest, right below my breast bone. It was difficult for me to look at the blazing red tissue when the nurse would clean it. That particular wound took months to close up. My left leg had scars as well, as the veins were taken from that part of my body to be used as a new artery to bypass my now diseased right coronary artery. My left thigh felt numb, tingly and painful when touched. I was told by my doctor that there was permanent nerve damage to that leg and I would have to learn to live with it. Fortunately for me, I have recovered some feeling in my left thigh, but it has taken years for it to recover, and it is still somewhat numb to the touch.

With each passing day in the RC I recognized that I was feeling more and more depressed. I would cry at the drop of a hat, had no hope, experienced acute anxiety, particularly at night, and felt terribly helpless. This was not the person I used to be before this horrific event.

My attending physician put in a request for a psychologist to talk with me. Good, I thought. This was what I did for a living so I was hopeful that this person would be someone I could turn to for some emotional support and understanding. Unfortunately, her visit did not turn out to be helpful at all. She stood by the doorway in my room, never taking a seat near my bed, seemingly in a hurry to get the session over with so that she could leave. Sensing her lack of empathy, I felt a coldness that was not consoling at all. The only thing she wanted to do was have me start on an antidepressant called Wellbutrin. After she left I felt even worse. She never returned to follow up to see how I was faring. Fortunately for me, my occupational therapist was just the opposite of the psychologist. She really listened and allowed me to have my feelings about what I was going through. I felt for the first time since my heart attack that someone was there who "really got it." You never know where your support is going to come from, and I think of her often for the blessing she was to me in my life at that point in time.

My physician took the advice of the psychologist and started me on the Wellbutrin. One of the side effects of this drug is to inhibit appetite. Now why was I put on a drug that would make my appetite even less than what it was? I had already lost a significant amount of weight, had NO appetite whatsoever, and now they were making it worse with this drug to treat my depression? This didn't make sense to me, so I had them discontinue it immediately.

Since my heart attack I have learned that depression is a very common side effect for cardiac patients.[3,4] The reasons are many. For those recovering from bypass surgery, like myself, the recovery is long and tedious, with a loss of strength and stamina that takes months to recover. Not being able to participate fully in life leaves a sadness that often turns into clinical depression. Patients who have stents inserted into their blocked coronary arteries have a much quicker physical recovery time but are left with a nagging fear and anxiety about when another artery will close up, requiring another intervention. And then there are those cardiac patients who live with a debilitating condition called angina, brought about because there is an inadequate supply of blood to the heart, resulting in pain in the chest, jaw, neck, back and arms. Nitroglycerin tablets are used often by these patients to dilate their constricted arteries to relieve the discomfort. Sitting still so as not to exert energy that causes the pain from angina becomes the new norm for those with this painful condition. No wonder we are all so depressed, waiting for the other shoe to drop.

Thankfully, the staff who cared for me in the RC understood why I was so depressed and could hold out hope for me, even though I was unable to believe at the time that things would eventually get better.

After about a week in the RC, I started to think about my psychotherapy clients that I had not been able to see since before Thanksgiving when my heart attack and surgery had taken place. I wanted to reach out to them to let them know what had happened to me. Most importantly, I wanted to reach the children I saw in my practice, many of whom had abandonment issues, to reassure them that I would be back to see them again when I was well. I actually got on the phone with one child in particular so that he would hear my voice and be reassured that I had not vanished for good. I was able to work on a letter while in rehab that I sent to all of my clients when I returned home, letting them know how I was doing and promising to inform them when I would be back at work and ready to reconvene our work together.

However, I felt as if I had let down all the people I had been helping. I felt useless and purposeless. I was so down and out that I didn't want to talk to friends or family much and spent my days basically alone. I do, however, remember the kindness of everyone who sent cards, flowers, and words of encouragement. A few came to visit with me but I was not very good company. On one occasion, my business partner and friend, Dawn, visited while I was in the occupational therapy room. She sat with me at my little table while I was stacking blocks, and the two of us had a good laugh as I was "doing my job." I must admit I became quite proficient in stacking those blocks. Being a Type A personality, I had to be the best block stacker ever!

Dale came to see me every day after work. He was exhausted and emotionally drained from the whole ordeal, but never missed spending time with me in the evenings. He later told me that he would go home, eat something quickly and finally fall into bed with our two cats and a heavy heart, only to repeat the same routine every day until the day I came home.

After two grueling weeks of rehabilitation, it was finally time for me to go home, but not before one last assignment by my physical therapist. She requested that we walk outdoors once around the building. Doing so seemed insurmountable to me at the time, and I curled up in my bed after lunch and cried and cried, not wanting to put forth that much physical effort, which I felt was in such short supply. She came to my room and saw me lying there in a heap of tears. She let me cry for a few minutes and then gently got me out of bed, into my tennis shoes, and out the door. We made our first walk around the perimeter of the building that day. I returned exhausted yet triumphant and hopeful that maybe, just maybe, one day I would be able to get back to my old life. I truly thanked her for her toughness conjoined with her kindness. At that time, it was the just the combination I needed to get myself moving forward in my recovery. When I went back to work months later and was feeling well again, I returned to the RC, found my physical therapist, and walked the whole length of the floor, doing my victory lap with both hands up in the air, just for her. I'll never forget the smile that crossed her face as she saw me in action, remembering the person I was when I left the RC and now seeing the fully functioning person I had once again become.

I couldn't wait to get home and sleep in my own bed for the first time in over a month.

5

Homecoming

It was now late December. My daughter, son, daughter-in-law and my 8-month-old grandson were in town to celebrate my homecoming. I remember leaving the RC, getting into our car and being driven home. Once there, I sat in a chair in our living room and watched all the activity around me. It seemed surreal to be home. I felt as though I was watching a movie that I wasn't even part of. It was also a bit unsettling not having the support of professional staff with me around the clock. In truth, I had an overwhelming fear that, left on my own, I would have another heart attack... and die.

The physical weakness continued. I couldn't pick up my sweet little grandson. I couldn't get myself into our tub. I had no energy to cook and still no desire to eat, but, even so, it was good to be home. My daughter and daughter-in-law carefully got me into the shower that first night so that I could feel clean and refreshed. They had purchased a bench seat for me to sit on as I couldn't stand for an extended period of time in the shower. My precious grandson brought a smile to my face and gave me the motivation to push on. I wanted to live to be able to see what kind of a person he would turn out to be.

Dale took a month off from work to be with me at home,

but that month quickly came to an end. I remember the first day I was on my own, fearful as to how I would be able to manage. To pass the time, I sat in a comfy chair in our bedroom with a stack of books. I can't remember another time in my life when I read so much. Throughout the day I would read and doze off, interspersed with brief walks in the hallway outside our condo and calls from friends and family. I didn't cook at all for over two months. Prior to my heart attack, cooking had been my passion, but even the prospect of turning on the oven was daunting. Thankfully, friends brought food to us over the course of the next two months, which I greatly welcomed and appreciated.

As the days went by I was still very depressed and in need of some treatment. My psychiatrist friend came to visit me shortly after my homecoming, and we discussed my worsening depression. She was able to prescribe the antidepressant Lexapro. I started on it the next day but had a terrible reaction. I was nauseous and couldn't eat or drink anything all day long. She then tried me on Remeron. This antidepressant is sometimes used with children who have cancer, and it works well to stimulate an appetite. The only other side effects that I experienced on this drug were weight gain (which I needed) and some initial drowsiness in the morning, which subsided within a week or two. I would take the pill at bedtime and sleep like a baby the whole night through.

Personally, I'm not a fan of pills, but being able to eat and sleep helped me recover from my depression. Thankfully, I was able to wean myself off the medication in six months.

Being a psychotherapist, I knew that my anxious psychological state was related to the traumatic events from my heart attack and bypass and aortic repair surgeries. I would relive in my mind the day I almost died, like a scene from a movie that kept playing repeatedly. I was having what is referred to as "flashbacks" from a condition called post-traumatic stress disorder, the illness that often strikes soldiers who have witnessed horrific events while in combat. It takes time and psychotherapy for the condition to improve. I sought the guidance of a psychotherapist to help me recover psychologically from what had happened to me. Seeking professional help from a licensed therapist is something I would highly recommend to anyone experiencing this kind of traumatic event.

A week after returning home I went to see my cardiologist for my first follow up visit. He advised me to participate in an outpatient Cardio Rehabilitation Program (CRP) at the hospital. I was still very weak and tremendously sad. Dale drove me there for my initial evaluation with one of the nurses on staff. She was a very young, perky nurse who greeted me and showed me around the facility. I was still very emotional and broke down in tears during our meeting. She didn't quite know how to respond to this sobbing woman as she nervously laughed and said, "Oh don't worry. You'll get better." She had no idea how I was feeling. After all, how could I get better feeling as lousy as I felt? Nonetheless, I was made to walk around the indoor track for twenty minutes, hooked up to a heart monitor to evaluate my heart function. I thought I was going to pass out after just a few laps. It felt as if they were telling me, "Go run a marathon." Upon arriving home after that ordeal, I slept the entire afternoon away.

The following week I reluctantly arrived for my first session. For the next 6 weeks, I would attend the CRP three times a week. Since Dale had returned to work full -time and I was still unable to drive, getting to rehab became a real challenge. Here's what I did. I relied on my problem-solving skills and ultimately came up with a plan. Remember the movie *Driving Miss Daisy*? Well, I sent an email to all my friends entitled, *Driving Miss Sherry*. And drive me they did for the next six weeks. It is often helpful to let others know what they can do to help you get you through your recovery and asking directly spells out exactly what is needed. Friends want to help. They just need to know what to do.

My routine at the CRP was 30 minutes of a cardio workout, followed by lifting light weights. One of the nurses would then give a 15-minute talk about some aspect of recovering from heart disease. Some of the lectures focused on nutrition. Program participants were advised to eat a diet low in fat, but one that could include small amounts of animal and dairy products. It was the very same information that my cardiologist had given me when I visited him in his office.

6

The Answer to Staying Alive

I was a very compliant patient until the day my sister, a nurse practitioner, recommended a book, *Prevent and Reverse Heart Disease,*[5] by Dr. Caldwell Esselstyn, Jr., a physician at the Cleveland Clinic.

Dr. Esselstyn was a world-renowned surgeon who had turned his interest away from surgery and towards the prevention and reversal of heart disease. The treatment was simple. He advised patients to adhere strictly to a whole foods, oil-free, plant-based diet (WFPD). That diet included fruits, vegetables, legumes and whole grains. To be avoided was "anything with a face." That meant no beef, poultry, pork or fish. He also advised patients to avoid dairy products, eggs, all oils, and even nuts, avocados and coconuts—all foods from the plant family that were high in fat.

Turning the pages of that book set in motion for me a series of events that would change my life forever. ***For the first time since my heart attack and surgery, a physician was telling me how, by following a relatively simple regimen, I could rid myself of heart disease forever.***

In his book, Dr. Esselstyn reported the health results of 17 critically ill heart patients who participated in his study. They had been seen by their cardiologists at The Cleveland Clinic and were told there was nothing more that could be done to treat their disease medically—no stents, no surgeries or new medications. Their options had run out. Their last resort was to participate in Dr. Esselstyn's study. These were patients who were desperate for any chance to survive.

The results of Dr. Esselstyn's study were first published in *The American Journal of Cardiology*[6] and were those results astounding! *After 12 years of strict adherence to his diet plan, not one of the study participants experienced a further cardiac event.* The message was clear: heart disease could be prevented and even reversed simply by changing one's diet.

Dr. Esselsytn reported substantially the same results in a 2013 study—this one involving 187 heart patients—conducted by him and his colleagues at The Cleveland Clinic Wellness Center and published in *The Journal of Family Practice.*[7] What we were learning from these two studies was that diet trumps genetics in the prevention and even reversal of heart disease. This was something directly contrary to what I had been told all along, namely, that my genetics predisposed me to this illness and that there was nothing much I could do to help myself.

Another pioneering physician, Dr. Dean Ornish, has been studying the effects of lifestyle changes on heart disease for 37 years. He has published numerous studies on the prevention and reversal of heart disease, and his results echo those of Esselstyn, all concluding that by adopting a WFPD, heart disease can be prevented and even reversed. One such study, published in 1998 in the *Journal of the American Medical Association* and entitled *Intensive Lifestyle Changes for Reversal of Coronary Heart Disease,*[8] informed physicians of the power of adopting a whole foods diet and other healthy lifestyle changes as a means of treating heart disease. A growing body of scientific evidence supporting this proposition continues to emerge. It truly is a hopeful time for heart patients, knowing that they have the ability to stop their disease dead in it tracks. Death from coronary artery disease is no longer inevitable.

In his book, Dr. Esselstyn shares the personal stories of

those patients he has treated with dietary intervention. One story that resonates with me was that of a surgeon at The Cleveland Clinic, Dr. Joe Crowe, who, in his 40's, had a sudden, near fatal heart attack. The location of his blockage precluded the placement of a stent and surgery was deemed too risky. He was in serious trouble, seemingly with no viable options. Desperate to live, he and his wife visited with the Esselstyns at their home and shared a plant-based meal with them. During dinner, Dr. Esselstyn and his wife Anne laid out the plan for how Dr. Crowe could treat his heart disease. Having nothing to lose and everything to gain, Dr. Crowe started on the Esselstyn plan the next day. Over the course of time there was clear evidence from his coronary angiograms that the blockage in his affected artery had receded so significantly as to no longer be of any concern. In short, he had reversed his heart disease.

Now one would think that cardiologists who read the results of these studies would be motivated to share them with their patients. That, however, is not what typically happens. Very few cardiologists inform patients of this life-saving regimen. I once asked a physician why this was so, and he told me one reason is that doctors don't always read the journals that publish this information. Amazingly, another doctor I had visited told me, "No one's going to make these kinds of dietary changes, and I don't have the time to explain all of this anyway."

In fairness to doctors, I continue to remind myself that they have spent years in medical school and residency programs training to treat the *symptoms* of heart disease. They were never given information about how a WFPD could *prevent* it in the first place. Instead, the accepted protocol was to prescribe medications to lower cholesterol and blood pressure levels along with procedures, such as stent insertions and bypass surgeries. These procedures were at best band-aid approaches that never addressed the root causes of heart disease and did nothing to prevent or reverse it.

As difficult as it is for me to say, I do believe that cardiologists might feel threatened by this new information for fear that their earning power would be reduced under our current insurance companies' reimbursement schedules if their patients used food over medicine and procedures to treat their heart disease. Undoubtedly, there is a great deal of money to be made by performing heart procedures and prescribing drugs, while there is little money to be made in prescribing fruits and vegetables. In other words, keeping patients teetering between sickness and health pretty much guarantees repeat business for these doctors.

What I want cardiologists to know is that I don't think they will end up in the poor house by telling us what the science knows about the power of whole foods to treat heart disease because not everyone will take their professional advice. There are, however, many of us who welcome this kind of good news and who are willing to make the necessary changes to take control of our disease. We deserve this life-saving information, and it is our doctors' ethical duty to deliver it to us. It is only then that we can decide for ourselves what we will do about our heart disease. To not inform patients, is, in my opinion, pure negligence.

On a positive note, Dr. Dean Ornish has worked diligently for well past a decade to convince Medicare to cover his program for reversing heart disease.[9] Medicare finally agreed and created a new benefit category called Intensive Cardiac Rehabilitation. Included in the 72-hour program are visits with a dietician to help patients transition to the WFPD, an exercise program, support, and stress reduction classes in yoga and meditation. While the reimbursements are peanuts (no pun intended) in comparison to cardiac procedures, it is at least a start.

Another promising development emerged at Kaiser Permanente Hospitals in California, where physicians are now required to tell their patients about how to promote their optimal heart health through a WFPD.[10]

Other efforts are underway to help individuals combat heart disease. For example, Dr. Esselstyn conducts all day seminars at The Cleveland Clinic instructing cardiac patients how to transition to the WFPD.[11] As well, Harvard Medical School has publicly acknowledged the benefits of eating a WFPD.[12] At the same time, many physicians and other healthcare providers are seeking training in lifestyle medicine to bring the message back to their patients that they can lead truly healthy lives by changing what they eat. Here are some other notable examples:

- Dr. John McDougall founded the Health and Medical Center in Santa Rosa, California, where he conducts training for healthcare providers and lay people about the WFPD. He also teaches medical students in several medical schools across the United States about lifestyle medicine and publishes a free online newsletter about the latest nutritional research findings.

- Dr. Neal Barnard created The Physicians Committee for Responsible Medicine in 1985, an advocacy and educational group that promotes the WFPD. In 2015, he opened The Barnard Medical Center in Washington, D.C., which provides complete primary care to patients using the WFPD model for the prevention and treatment of many chronic western illnesses such as heart disease, diabetes, certain cancers and autoimmune diseases.

- Dr. Pamela Popper established The Wellness Forum, an organization in Columbus, Ohio, that educates and trains healthcare providers and the lay community in how to maximize health by eating the WFPD. Dr. Popper produces bi-weekly videos on the latest research on important healthcare topics and disseminates the information in an understandable format to her listeners.

- Dr. T. Colin Campbell has been researching the benefits

of the WFPD as a nutritional biochemist for his entire career and, in addition to publishing his well-known work, *The China Study*, and hundreds of articles in respected scientific journals, he offers a certification program for healthcare providers and the lay public in plant-based nutrition through the T. Colin Campbell Center for Nutritional Studies in collaboration with e-Cornell.

- Dr. Michael Greger disseminates nutritional research findings through free articles and videos offered through his nutritionfacts.org website.

- And, finally, and most encouraging, in 2017, the American Medical Association (AMA) issued a policy statement to remove disease-causing foods from hospital menus nationwide. "AMA hereby call on US hospitals to improve the health of patients, staff, and visitors by providing a variety of healthful food," the AMA's resolution states, "including plant-based meals and meals that are low in fat, sodium, and added sugars." This statement also asks hospitals and staff to lead by example by "eliminating processed meats from menus and providing and promoting healthful beverages."[13]

So, it seems that things are changing, albeit slowly. Many healthcare professionals are now being advised to use food over medicine in their treatment plans, thereby helping patients stay out of their offices because they are finally able to stop and reverse not only heart disease but also type 2 diabetes, some cancers and many autoimmune diseases.

With the research supporting the findings of Dr. Esselstyn and Dr. Ornish, pharmaceutical companies are no doubt getting very nervous. They know that if patients tried food over drugs to treat their conditions that their sales would surely decline. Make no doubt about it, big pharma will do anything to continue to encourage doctors to prescribe heart and blood pressure medications as a first line of defense against heart diseases. Why? Because these two classes of drugs represent huge profits for these companies.

What I want to be clear about though is that for some people, including myself, some of these medications are necessary. Even while eating a WFPD, I still struggle with high blood pressure no matter what I have done to reduce it, including significantly lowering my sodium intake, eating many leafy greens, beans, fruits and vegetables, and drinking hibiscus tea (known to help lower blood pressure). I have also tried to get off of my cholesterol-lowering medication but have seen that when I do, for some reason, my LDL goes way up (past a point of safety for me) as does my overall cholesterol. I have found that by taking only 5mg of my Crestor every day, I am able to keep my total cholesterol around 130 and my "bad" LDL cholesterol around 60 (anything below 80 is considered excellent). I can live with taking small doses of meds to lower my blood pressure and cholesterol so long as I do not have significant side effects from them, which I don't.

When I tell others about what I have done with my diet to prevent any more heart disease I am often asked "But what is the science behind this diet, and how does it work?" This is a very important question, and one that needs to be understood. Let me try to share with you, in layman's terms, what I have learned about heart disease from Dr. Esselstyn and Dr. Ornish and from my own coursework at the T. Colin Campbell Center for Nutritional Studies, where in 2012 I received my certificate in plant-based nutrition.

Our vascular health depends on two very important factors. The first has to do with endothelial cells, which line every artery in our body. Healthy endothelial cells mean our artery linings remain slippery and smooth, allowing blood to flow effortlessly throughout the body. Secondly, if we have arteries with healthy endothelial cells, our bodies can produce a gas called nitric oxide, which acts as a natural dilator within our arteries. This is very important for the heart as our heart muscle depends upon receiving adequate blood flow to provide it with enough oxygen and nutrients to pump blood efficiently throughout our bodies. When we eat animal and dairy products, as well as processed oils, we build up a sticky substance called plaque on the lining of our arteries. This plaque buildup then damages the endothelial cells, which in turn inhibits the production of nitric oxide. This continual, gradual buildup of plaque within our arteries sets the stage for coronary artery disease.

So, what role does this plaque buildup play during a heart attack? First, we must distinguish between two different types of plaque. The first type of plaque is older and has been sitting within our arteries for quite some time. It is composed mainly of calcium and scar tissue and does not pose the biggest risk for heart attacks. Less than 15% of all heart attacks are caused by this older plaque closing off a coronary artery.[14]

The more worrisome plaques are the newer, fatty ones that account for approximately 87% of heart attacks. Why is this so? Here's what happens. When blood is rushing past a newer plaque, it may rupture the very thin, fibrous cap sitting on top of the plaque, spilling the pussy substance into the artery where the rupture occurred. When this happens a whole set of events is set in motion that can lead to a heart attack. The body naturally wants to repair that rupture so it goes to work trying to form a clot over it, just as when we cut a finger and the clotting process stops our finger from continuing to bleed. Unfortunately, in the vessels leading up to the heart, this clotting may work too well, and, in some cases, may close the entire artery off where the clot has formed. When this happens, blood cannot reach the heart muscle, and a part of the heart dies from a lack of oxygen and nutrients. For some, this means instantaneous death. For those who survive, that part of the heart muscle that was deprived of adequate blood weakens and scars, and if there are multiple heart attacks, the heart may eventually fail. This condition is called congestive heart failure.

The less dangerous, older plaques do not rupture as do the newer plaques and may be detectable through angiograms. Newer plaques, however, can develop at any time and may not be known to patient or doctor until it is too late. So, the only way to prevent plaque from building up within our arteries is to refrain from eating the foods that cause it to form in the first place. Those foods, as mentioned previously, are oils of any kind, chicken, beef, pork, fish, eggs, and dairy products.

So, what do I eat, you might be asking? I eat everything that grows in the ground, including a wide variety of vegetables, fruits, whole grains and legumes, and I have found ways to prepare them that are tasty and filling.

It is important to understand that plant foods do not contain cholesterol, which can be found only in animal foods. Anytime our total cholesterol levels rise above 150, we are putting ourselves at risk for a heart attack. The "bad" LDL cholesterol must remain below 80 and our triglycerides below 150. To be sure, our bodies do need cholesterol, but what many do not know is that we produce just the right amounts of cholesterol within our bodies. Eating foods that contain cholesterol actually signals the body to produce even more cholesterol. So you see the cycle. Getting off the detrimental cholesterol merry-go-round can be done only with a WFPD, and, in some cases, a cholesterol-lowering medication. However, relying on medication alone is not enough; it is only a WFPD that will provide you with the insurance policy you need to prevent and even reverse your heart disease.

As was mentioned earlier, Dr. Esselstyn even advocates that those with known heart disease eliminate certain plant foods such as nuts, avocados and coconuts because of their high fat content. While I understand that these foods are high in fat, a more recent study from Dean Ornish indicates that nuts may have a protective effect against heart disease.[15] What is most important for me is to eat whole foods, including small amounts of some nuts and avocados. I discussed this with Dr. T. Colin Campbell at the Plant-based Cooking Summit that I attended in 2016, and he agreed that these plant foods are acceptable in small amounts. Further research will clarify the salutary effects of these whole foods.

I am often asked three questions about my new diet. One is, "Why can't you eat what has been termed heart healthy olive oil?" Well, according to the work of Dr. Esselstyn, Dr. Ornish and many other well-known physicians and researchers, *all* oils, including olive oil, are full of saturated fat, contain no nutritional value and constitute highly processed foods. What is surprising to many is that olive oil contains 11-14% of this fat, the same artery-clogging fat that is present in a slice of roast beef![16] I am doing everything I can to keep my arteries healthy, so I avoid all oils, even olive oil.

Let me tell you about one important study, conducted in Colombia by Dr. Linda Carney, on ten healthy young volunteers,[17] which may help you better understand the effects of oils on our arterial system. In this study, subjects were fed potato soup that had added to it 60ml of either olive oil, soybean oil or palm oil that was either fresh or had been used for frying 10 or 20 times. The effects of these different oils were measured by performing a flow-mediated vasodilation on the study subjects while they fasted and again three hours after the soup meal. Blood samples were taken as well at the same time.

Here's what was found. Endothelial function (the ability of the arteries to expand as a response to nitric oxide) decreased 32% and triglycerides went up 27% after ingesting these oils. The adverse effects were observed with all three kinds of oil tested, both fresh or fried. Dr. Carney has posted other research results on her site that confirm the same results for all oils. So, the bottom line on this subject is to leave the oils on the shelf in the store. They are not health foods.

The second question I am often asked is "Where do you get your protein?" We have been so conditioned to think that protein equates with animal foods that most people are unaware that fruits, vegetables, whole grains, and legumes all contain protein, in just the right amounts that our bodies require. All the animal industries (beef, poultry, fish, pork, dairy) play the "protein card" to encourage us to eat their products. Remember the milk campaign, "Milk Does a Body Good?" Well, actually, milk does just the opposite, with the main protein in milk, casein, having been found to be a known carcinogen.[18] Further, the fat in milk (even skim milk) introduces cholesterol into our bloodstream, which will eventually lay plaque in our arteries. (To learn more about casein and its carcinogenic effects, I recommend you read *The China Study* by Dr. T. Colin Campbell. In his research with rats he was able to show that he could "turn on" or "turn off" cancerous tumor growth, depending on the levels of casein delivered to the rats in their diet.)

In addition to eating the wrong type of protein, Americans consume too much of it for optimal health. Eating plants provides us with about 10% of our daily calories in the form of protein, the amount that we need to keep us alive and well.[19] In contrast, animal proteins introduce fat and cholesterol into our system and are the main reason that 36% of Americans have heart disease.

The third question I am frequently asked is "Isn't it hard to give up animal foods?" The short answer is no. You see, if I were to eat them, I would surely have more heart disease in my future. My life is too precious for me to even consider going back to eating the very foods that caused my heart disease in the first place. Having my chest cut open one time was enough for me. I never want to be back on that operating table, and I'll do whatever it takes to avoid that scenario. Gone are the days of leaving the table after a big meal feeling stuffed and sluggish.

Instead, I feel satisfied and energetic. Yes, it took time to learn a new way of preparing food, but it was easy in comparison to my recovery from my heart attack and bypass surgery. And nowadays there are groups to join of like-minded people who will support you in your transition to this new way of eating, a transition that is facilitated by an abundance of free resources easily accessible on the web.

Some final observations:

- After I finished Dr. Esselstyn's book, I watched the documentary *Forks Over Knives* and read *The China Study*, by Dr. T. Colin Campbell. What I learned about heart disease from Dr. Campbell's study was eye-opening. In parts of rural China where people ate a mainly WFPD, heart disease rarely existed.[20] How interesting.

- And this pattern was found in other parts of the world. For example, in Norway, during World War II, the population survived mainly on plants since the Germans removed their access to animal foods when food rationing occurred. The result? Heart disease rates dropped dramatically during those war years, only to rise once the war ended, with people once again eating animal and dairy products on a regular basis.[21]

- I have also learned that the Papua Highlanders of New Guinea have no coronary artery disease because their diet consists of nineteen varieties of sweet potatoes, even though they are heavy smokers. They do, however, have high rates of lung disease.[22]

So, the answer, in short, is nutrition. There is no medical procedure or pill that can prevent or reverse heart disease. All they can do is treat symptoms. Moving away from the standard American diet to a WFPD will save your life. It did mine.

7

Finding A Just Right Cardiologist In Houston

ollowing my heart attack, with all my newly acquired information, I visited the cardiologist that had handled my failed catherization. With Dr. Esselstyn's book in hand, I was eager to share with him what I had learned. To my utter surprise he told me he knew nothing about Dr. Esselstyn or his initial study at the Cleveland Clinic. He casually flipped through the pages, stopping to examine some photographs of angiograms. While my doctor noted the improvement in the coronary arteries of the patients shown by this study, he had no interest in talking to me about its implications for my own treatment. Since I had already started on the WFPB, I decided that I wanted a cardiologist who knew about the importance of treating heart disease by this means. In short, this doctor was clearly not the right one for me.

If prior to my heart attack a physician had told me about the possibility that I could have protected myself from heart disease by changing my diet, I would hope that I would have listened and had made changes a long time ago. But no one did. I am not alone. The majority of U.S. physicians receive little or no training in nutrition in medical school. And when physicians do talk about it, it is not discussed in terms of disease prevention. The majority still are of the view that eating animal foods and dairy products are just fine choices "in moderation." Unfortunately, moderation of these foods will eventually lead to heart disease for many.

Furthermore, traditionally trained nutritionists are likewise of little help. They continue to advocate a diet that is rich in animal products. Why, I kept asking myself, are these practitioners not telling us about what the science teaches about preventing and reversing heart disease through lifestyle changes?

On my quest to find a doctor whose views were compatible with mine, I made an appointment to see a doctor at one of Houston's most prestigious medical centers. I told her my story and what I had learned from Dr. Esselstyn. She at least was aware of his work but was still advising her patients to eat the Mediterranean diet, one that is rich in fruits, vegetables, legumes, nuts and whole grains but also includes animal products (eggs, chicken, fish and some beef and pork), along with olive oil. In fact, she was currently doing cooking demonstrations at a local grocery store using olive oil, promoting it as "heart healthy." I had a conversation with her about this at one of my visits. She still believed that olive oil was good for the heart, and while she supported me in my no-oil diet, she continued to recommend the Mediterranean diet to her patients.

Finally, I found a cardiologist in Texas, Dr. Baxter Montgomery, who had the same views about nutrition as I did. He founded the Montgomery Wellness Center, where patients like me could receive treatment for their heart disease through plant-based nutrition. One of the most exciting aspects of his clinic was an on-site cafe, where I would often stop to eat lunch after my appointment. A fabulous chef created some marvelous no-oil, plant-based foods that I was able to enjoy. What a relief it was to finally be with a doctor who was practicing medicine by using whole foods as the first line of defense against heart disease.

Sadly though, Dr. Montgomery is the exception to the rule. What I advise people to do when selecting a cardiologist (or an internist) is to find someone who at least understands and supports what you are doing and who does not think that drugs and procedures should be your first step in treatment. Ultimately it is up to each of us to educate our doctors by showing them how well we do when eating this way. Maybe one day, they will start telling patients about the miraculous results that can be obtained by eating the WFPD. And if your doctor doesn't support you in your efforts, find another doctor.

The same goes for a nutritionist. Recognize that the majority of nutritionists are trained to teach people to eat animal products (although they will tell you to make low fat choices) as part of a daily nutritional plan. Keep looking until you find a nutritionist who is trained in plant-based nutrition. They are out there.

8

From Patient to Educator:
Getting the Word Out

After my near-death experience, I was determined to share with others all that I had learned in my journey back to health. So, I asked my cardiologist at the time (the one who was promoting the Mediterranean diet) about becoming a volunteer at her hospital. My purpose, I told her, was to educate others about the benefits of eating an oil-free WFPD. She put me in touch with the volunteer coordinator, and, shortly thereafter, I began attending the hospital's orientation training. What happened during that orientation still makes me shake my head in dismay to this day.

On the first day of training, I was given a tour of the hospital by its public relations director. Our first stop was to an area that resembled a museum. There were displays everywhere you turned chronicling the history of the treatment of heart disease in that institution. I must admit it was fascinating to see some of the old devices that had been used to treat patients years ago. To be sure, we have come a long way since those early pioneering days. Nevertheless, what was conspicuously absent was any mention of nutrition in fighting this disease.

Our next stop was to a surgical suite. There I observed a fairly large man lying on the operating table with his chest cut wide open as his surgeon performed open heart bypass surgery. I felt sick to my stomach watching this, as that had been me on that table in the not too distant past. At that moment, I felt traumatized all over again. I sat down and turned my head away from the operating table. It was just too difficult for me to watch. My cardiologist was supposed to have joined us at this point in our orientation, but she got caught up with a patient and could not steel herself away. It probably would have been a good idea to have had her there. I'm not sure what purpose it served to have me watch this surgery, as it didn't relate to what I had proposed to do in my volunteer role.

We were then taken to the hospital's animal lab where I saw a cow with an artificial heart walking on a treadmill. All I wanted to do was to reach out and comfort that poor animal. The hospital took great pride in its research in developing a mechanical heart. All I felt, however, was profound sadness for that beautiful cow being used in this experimentation, knowing that she would die within a few weeks when the experiment concluded. There had to be a better way to test devices, one that did not entail using animals in this way. Thank goodness for the Physicians Committee For Responsible Medicine, which is working assiduously to prevent any kind of animal experimentation.

And, finally, we entered a lab of a hospital scientist who was actually making a new heart in a test tube! Very fascinating stuff, but I kept wondering to myself, what about nutrition? What about preventing the need for all this in the first place by teaching people how to avoid heart disease?

I couldn't help but ask this question of the director of public relations. His reaction at first was a blank stare. When he finally did speak he said, "No, we aren't involved in that type of research." I was starting to get it. What I thought was the most important research they could be undertaking was not even on their radar screen. It soon became evident to me that the path I was about to embark upon—educating others about heart disease prevention through proper nutrition—was hardly going to be an easy one. To the contrary, I was in for a rather bumpy ride.

The final step in the orientation process was a grocery tour led by two of the hospital's nutritionists. I dutifully followed them through the aisles and listened to them talk about a heart healthy diet. I couldn't believe what they were saying. One started talking about olive oil and how good it was for the heart. I asked her "Are you aware of the research out of the Cleveland Clinic about how olive oil inhibits the production of nitric oxide in our arteries, damaging the endothelial cells that line our arteries, which can lead to heart disease?" She looked at me as though I was from another planet and insisted that olive oil was a healthy oil and good for heart health.

But the worst was yet to come. Once in the meat department, the nutritionist actually said that heart patients could have bacon "once in a while" because we shouldn't deprive ourselves of everything we loved. Ok, we were in Texas, but come on! Now I was not only shocked but furious that such advice was being given by a nutritionist! This world-renowned hospital in Houston, Texas, was not a place showing any awareness about the value of a WFPD and certainly would not welcome having a patient talk about it with other heart patients. As I was leaving the grocery tour, one of the nutritionists approached me and said, "If we have a patient interested in how you eat, maybe you could talk to them about it?" While that was a nice invitation, I felt it was her job to become educated on this subject so that she could give them this information herself. It was after this tour that I decided that I was not comfortable doing volunteer work for this hospital and immediately withdrew from their program.

I have never been one to give up. Even with my growing

frustration with the medical community, I devised another plan to get the word out. I decided to approach those kind nurses with whom I had worked in the CRP and asked them if I could present some information on Dr. Esselstyn's prevention and reversal program in all eight of their cardio rehabilitation classes during the educational segment of their program. I also offered to bring a sampling of some of my food to each class. They enthusiastically agreed to let me talk to their patients.

For the next two weeks, I spoke to all the CRP groups, reaching well over 100 patients. I told them how, since starting on my diet, my cholesterol had fallen from 175 down to 105 in about three months and my LDL cholesterol had dropped to 48. I shared with them the foods I ate and a little bit about the science behind the diet revealed in Dr. Esselstyn's work. We talked about how getting total cholesterol below 150 and "bad" LDL cholesterol below 80 was imperative in order to heart attack-proof oneself. The response was heartwarming. After each of my talks I could see faces light up and hope start to build. Many came up to me after my talk and thanked me for telling them what I had learned. I heard over and over again that they had never been given this information before and were as baffled as I had been as to why. I know that many purchased Dr. Esselstyn's book and embarked on this path. I can't tell you how good it felt to finally be able to share with others what I had learned. Interestingly, there was only one man in all of the groups I presented to who didn't like my message and actually got angry, telling me, "I'm not giving up meat. I love meat!" Sadly, he's a shining example of why cardiologists will never be put out of business.

As a result of presenting this new information at the CRP classes, I was invited by the nursing staff to speak to the hospital's Mended Hearts group. This group met once a month for the purpose of providing heart patients education on heart disease and to provide support. Welcomed by a standing room only crowd, I presented my talk, entitled "How To Heart

Attack-Proof Yourself With a Whole Foods, No-Oil, Plant-based Diet." It explored the work of Dr. Esselstyn and others in the field. I think this title may have caught their attention! I had brought along about 20 copies of Dr. Esselstyn's book to sell at cost, which sold out in minutes! People were hungry for this information, information that they had never received from their own cardiologists.

What I found very disconcerting at that meeting, however, was what the hospital served these cardiac patients for dinner that night. They had their choice of cold cut sandwiches, tuna salad, fruits and vegetables (yeah!) and cookies and cakes for dessert. I mentioned to the audience when I finished my talk what I had observed about their dinner on the buffet table, asking them to please ask for foods in the future that would help them heal from their disease rather than progress it. I said this rather tongue in cheek, but I think they got the message.

At the conclusion of my presentation I provided a signup sheet for those interested in meeting once a month for a pot luck dinner to help them transition to this new way of eating. Because the sign-up sheet quickly filled up, I asked the nurses to request a room from the hospital for these meetings. Guess what happened? We were turned down! The nurses who had helped me get the word out were told this was not going to be sponsored by the hospital. I even wrote to my surgeon to ask for help, but I never got a response. Once again, another door shut. What was happening here? What were they afraid of?

I've already discussed my own thoughts as to what they feared. It is difficult to say this, but in the end, I do believe that it comes down to dollars and cents. Hospitals depend on expensive heart procedures and surgeries to keep them afloat, and a cardiologist will receive far greater reimbursement for placing a stent in a blocked coronary artery and a surgeon for doing a bypass than he or she ever would for providing nutritional counseling. Something has to change.

Speaking about big money, the total cost of my surgery and hospital stay approached a million dollars. I was fortunate that our insurance covered most of it. The psychological costs were high as well. I had missed four months of work and had become depressed and anxious. It took months for these conditions to improve. Until I met Dr. Baxter Montgomery, I had no guidance about the life-saving nature of the WFPD and had to educate myself.

When I went back to work, I had to do so gradually, seeing only a few clients a day until I felt I had the strength to do more. Some of my clients stuck with me after my four-month absence, while others needed help while I was gone and switched therapists. In a way, I was back to square one in having to rebuild my practice. It was an exhausting time, but within nine months after my heart attack, I felt pretty normal again. Nine months, however, is a long recovery period. It was during my recovery that I began to realize that I had to take life at a much slower pace. The drive within me needed to be tempered, and I listened to that inner voice that advised me to take it down a notch.

One way that I learned to move through my life with more calm and ease was to practice yoga. I had started my yoga journey with my teacher and dear friend, Ceily Levy, when we lived in Chicago. She taught me how to live life in the present moment, how to breathe deeply and slowly, and how to work at calming the mind through the practice of yoga. This changed my life for the better just as much as did my change in diet. I never found a yoga teacher in Houston who inspired me as much as Ceily, so I took to practicing on my own every day while living there. I would go to an outdoor area to practice my yoga poses, finishing with meditation and then giving thanks for being alive each and every day. Gratitude became both my new mantra and an integral part of my healing process.

Meanwhile, my close friend and work colleague, Dawn Nelson, decided to join me in eating a WFPD. Having kept a vigil while I was in the hospital, she saw firsthand the ravages of heart disease and decided she wanted to do something for herself to avoid this ever happening to her. This led to us experimenting in our kitchens, cooking up lots of new things that we would bring to work and taste test together. Dawn thought it was important to present what we had learned at the *Hope and Healing Center* in Houston. This center had just opened (at former President George H.W. Bush's church), and Dawn and I put together a proposal to teach a class there that we called *Staying Alive—An Introduction to Plant-based Living*.

The class was a huge success. About 25 people participated, three of whom were nurses from the CRP that I had attended. Dawn and I presented the various reasons why eating this way was good for our bodies and how it could prevent many of our western diseases, such as heart disease, some cancers, stroke, type 2 diabetes and many of our autoimmune diseases. The best part of the class though was the smorgasbord of whole foods Dawn and I had prepared, which the class had an opportunity to sample. They couldn't believe how delicious everything tasted—and without a drop of oil!

I began to see within myself the possibility of changing the way Americans eat, one person at a time, by presenting these types of classes. An opportunity arose shortly thereafter that allowed me to reach a broader audience. I had been watching TV one day and came across a local program called *Women Who Lead*. This show, hosted by a local pastor, Dr. Ruth Olison, invited women to talk about what they were doing to make a difference in their communities. It was a half hour show so there was ample opportunity to go into depth about the subjects being discussed.

I wrote to Dr. Olison, telling her about my experience with heart disease and what I was doing to educate others on the benefits of the WFPD. I was pleasantly surprised when she extended to me an invitation to be on her show.

I had never done a TV show before and was quite nervous yet excited at the same time. I think I handled myself fairly well. Having performed in many plays and musicals during high school, in front of large audiences, was definitely helpful to me that day. I told my story and explained why the WFPD was the best course for heart patients to heal themselves often without the need for pills or procedures. At the end of the show I presented Dr. Olison with my banana bread, a recipe from Ann Esselstyn (Dr. Esselstyn's wife) that appeared in *Prevent and Reverse Heart Disease*. She and her staff couldn't believe it was made without eggs and without any oil. I wrote to Ann Esselstyn to let her know about the show and how well her banana bread had been received. She and Dr. Esselstyn watched the show that morning and, later that day, Dr. Esselstyn phoned to thank me for talking about what I had learned and for continuing to spread the word.

I think it was at that moment that I realized that I had found a new purpose for my life. I would use my energy to educate others about the prevention and reversal of heart disease. I knew there would be many more hurdles to overcome, but the importance of the message far outweighed any obstacles that might lie in my path.

9

Institutional Misinformation

One of the most difficult challenges I have faced in my efforts to inform Americans about the dangers of the standard American diet (known by the all too fitting acronym, SAD) has to do with messages coming from, among others, our government and the American Heart Association, two places where Americans often look for nutritional guidance. In January 2016 the United States Department of Agriculture (USDA), along with the Department of Health and Human Services (DHHS), issued guidelines for what Americans should be eating for optimal health (the Guidelines). The Guidelines, which will remain in effect until 2020, are disturbing at best and life-threatening at worst.

An example of how misguided the Guidelines are is the omission of any mention of concern over cholesterol, which we know contributes to the development of heart disease. Because of this exclusion from the Guidelines, on January 6, 2016, the Physicians Committee for Responsible Medicine (PCRM), Dr. John McDougall, and other well respected California-based physicians filed suit in the US District Court (North District of California) against the USDA and the DHHS over the position of the Department of Guidelines Advisory Committee

(DGAC) "that cholesterol is no longer a nutrient of concern for overconsumption."[23]

This position resulted from a 20-year campaign by the egg industry to dispel the notion that eggs are a major contributor of coronary artery disease, despite the fact that it is the number one cause of death in the United States.

The "Complaint for Declarative and Injunctive Relief," as it was fashioned, while not leading to a change in the Guidelines themselves, resulted in the inclusion of the following statement that accompanied the Guidelines, which were released on January 7, 2016:

"The Key Recommendation from the 2010 Dietary Guidelines to limit consumption of dietary cholesterol to 300 mg per day is not included in the 2015 edition, but this change does not suggest that dietary cholesterol is no longer important to consider when building healthy eating patterns. As recommended by the IMO (Institute of Medicine), individuals should eat as little dietary cholesterol as possible while consuming a healthy eating pattern. Strong evidence from mostly prospective cohort studies, but also randomized controlled trials, has shown that eating patterns that include lower intake of dietary cholesterol are associated with reduced risk of CVD (cardiovascular disease), and moderate evidence indicates that these eating patterns are associated with reduced risk of obesity."[24]

Very interesting indeed. Now take a look at the foods that our government recommends Americans eat as part of their "healthy eating pattern."

The Guidelines

A healthy eating pattern includes:

- A variety of vegetables from all of the subgroups—

dark green, red and orange, legumes (beans and peas), starchy, and other

- Fruits, especially whole fruits
- Grains, at least half of which are whole grains
- Fat-free or low-fat dairy, including milk, yogurt, cheese, and/or fortified soy beverages
- A variety of protein foods, including seafood, lean meats and poultry, eggs, legumes (beans and peas), and nuts, seeds, and soy products
- Oils

A healthy eating pattern is characterized by:

- limited saturated fats and trans fats, added sugars, and sodium
- Consumption of less than 10 percent of calories per day from added sugars
- Consumption of less than 10 percent of calories per day from saturated fats
- Consumption of less than 2,300 milligrams (mg) per day of sodium

To me, the Guidelines are appalling. They guarantee that Americans who eat what the USDA recommends are at great risk for developing diabetes, heart disease, some cancers and many autoimmune diseases. And for those of us with heart disease who adhere to these guidelines, we will surely watch our disease progress. Many will die needlessly as well, leaving wives, husbands, children, grandchildren, relatives and dear friends behind. It need not be this way. The USDA should recommend what the science has been telling us for years—that by eating a WFPD we can avoid getting these diseases. Since the USDA won't tell you the truth, know it for yourself, and adopt a diet that will allow you to avoid these diseases.

Following the USDA's Guidelines throughout my life almost cost me my life. No more. I know better now.

So, the question remains, "Why is the government recommending foods that the science is clearly telling us will cause disease rather than prevent it?" The answer lies in the powerful lobbyists who represent the animal industries. They spend enormous amounts of money advertising their products and lobbying those who make the decisions for the Guidelines. They will do anything to keep the truth from the American public in order to maximize industry profits.

Much of the research the USDA bases its recommendations on comes from studies funded by the meat, poultry, pork and dairy industries.[25] It's hard to be neutral when the scientists producing the research findings are getting paid by the very industries they are studying. Science is supposed to be unbiased, and it is outrageous that any study would be considered such when it is paid for by the industries that want us to continue to buy their products. Looking out for our health? I think not.

It is also important to note that the National Institutes of Health (NIH), our nation's medical research agency, which is part of the U.S. Department of Health and Human Services, claims that they are making important discoveries that improve health and save lives. However, there exists no Nutrition Institute among the 27 existing Institutes under its umbrella.

Watching Nelson Campbell's documentary PlantPure Nation, one sees firsthand the influence of animal industry lobbyists on a legislative body that had an opportunity to issue a proclamation that stated that an oil-free, whole foods, plant-based diet is the optimal diet for health. It was defeated, albeit narrowly, mainly because there was fear that in voting for it, animal industry lobbyists would withdraw financial support for these legislators in future elections. While some understood the importance of the proclamation, to have voted for it would have meant political suicide.

Another powerful organization that advises us on how to treat our heart disease is The American Heart Association (AHA). I, like most Americans, always thought that the AHA had the latest information about heart disease and that they would of course disseminate it to the public. Boy was I wrong. Here's what I learned when I volunteered for them as a speaker in their public education department.

During their orientation program, I learned how they felt volunteers could help fight against heart disease. They were kind enough to provide us with lunch, or so I thought, until I saw what was on the buffet table. Once again (just like at the Mended Hearts Group event), I saw cold cuts, potato chips, some fresh fruits and veggies (yeah again!) and a plate full of big old cookies! Was I ever glad that I had packed my lunch that day. I could't believe my eyes. If it were't so tragically unhealthy and dangerous for heart patients, it would be comical. What was happening here? This organization that was charged with helping people prevent heart disease was serving it up on the lunch table!

As part of their speaker division, I was told to look for speaking opportunities on their website. Not one organization had requested a speaker on plant-based nutrition. I was not that surprised, however, knowing that the AHA promotes the Mediterranean diet for those with heart disease. This diet includes fruits, vegetables, whole grains, low fat dairy products, skinless poultry, fish, nuts, legumes and non-tropical vegetable oils, such as canola oil, olive oil, peanut oil, sesame oil and vegetable oil. They refer to these oils as being "heart healthy" oils, even though, as mentioned earlier, olive oil is 11-14% saturated fat—the same artery-clogging fat that is found in beef. I knew from my own research that while this diet, endorsed by the AHA, may slow the progression of heart disease, it would not prevent or reverse it.[26] Once again I found myself uncomfortable volunteering for an organization that did not advocate for the most current and relevant, life-saving scientific information on the prevention and reversal of heart disease.

To better understand how the AHA came to their current recommendations regarding diet and heart disease, I decided to read about its goals and philosophy. Below is their official statement from their website, together with my reactions.[27]

Who We Are

The American Heart Association is the nation's oldest and largest voluntary organization dedicated to fighting heart disease and stroke. Founded by six cardiologists in 1924, our organization now includes more than 22.5 million volunteers and supporters. We fund innovative research, fight for stronger public health policies, and provide critical tools and information to save and improve lives. Our nationwide organization includes 156 local offices and more than 3,000 employees. We moved our national headquarters from New York to Dallas in 1975 to be more centrally located. The American Stroke Association was created as a division in 1997 to bring together the organization's stroke-related activities.

What We Do

To improve the lives of all Americans, we provide public health education in a variety of ways. We're the nation's leader in CPR education training. We help people understand the importance of healthy lifestyle choices. We provide science-based treatment guidelines to healthcare professionals to help them provide quality care to their patients. We educate lawmakers, policymakers and the public as we advocate for changes to protect and improve the health of our communities. Our volunteer experts select scientific research most worthy of funding—with great results. The association has funded more than $3.8 billion in heart disease and stroke research, more than any organization outside the federal government.

My response: Since the AHA states that its goal is to improve the lives of all Americans, I would ask it to fund a prospective randomized trial that would compare the reduction in heart attacks, strokes and death for patients who eat a Mediterranean diet versus those who consume a no-oil WFPD. We already have two large prospective randomized trials comparing the Mediterranean diet with the westernized diet that influence the guidelines, showing a 30% (PREDIMED)[28] to 39% (HALE)[29] reduction in heart attack, stroke and death compared with a westernized diet. These results are horrendous when we recognize that there is a 70% persistence rate! They make it imperative that we push forward with research that supports the data we already have from longitudinal studies that show much better results with a WFPD. Only then will physicians find it impossible to continue to ignore results.

Why We're Needed

Heart disease is the No. 1 killer in the world. Stroke ranks second globally and is a leading cause of severe disability. Too many families are losing loved ones of all ages. Each year, these diseases kill more than 786,000 Americans, which is larger than the population of several states (Alaska, North Dakota, Vermont and Wyoming). Some form of cardiovascular disease affects more than one in every three adult Americans. Many suffer terribly from disabilities caused by these diseases. The American Heart Association wants everyone to understand the threat—and to know that cardiovascular diseases and stroke are largely preventable. Risks can be lowered by adhering to what we call Life's Simple 7: not smoking, being physically active, maintaining a healthy body weight, eating a healthy diet, controlling blood pressure, controlling cholesterol and controlling blood sugar.

My response: How are we maintaining a healthy body weight, controlling cholesterol and blood sugar with the foods you serve at your own volunteer training? Cold cuts, potato chips and cookies are doing just the opposite. You say that heart disease is largely preventable (and I agree), yet, with the foods you are promoting you continue to keep people sick enough to need drugs and interventions. Going to your Go Red Cookbook,[30] one finds animal-based products and olive oil as standard fare. Indeed, one recipe endorsed by the AHA, Turkey Medallions, calls for one pound of turkey cutlets along with olive oil. We know that the cholesterol in turkey and the fat in olive oil will contribute to plaque buildup in our arteries even in small amounts, with a cumulative effect over our lifetimes that will ultimately cause coronary artery disease in at least 36% of Americans. Not acceptable in my book.

Our 2020 Goal

We are working toward improving the cardiovascular health of all Americans by 20 percent, and reducing deaths from cardiovascular diseases and stroke by 20 percent, all by the year 2020.

My response: Not good enough. If this disease is largely preventable, why not aim to reduce it by 100%? The AHA could be doing so much more to eliminate this disease by promoting what the science tells us: eating a whole foods oil-free plant-based diet. I encourage everyone to challenge the AHA's year 2020 goal and to demand that they start telling the public the truth about the research of Dr. Esselstyn and Dr. Dean Ornish, research that unequivocally demonstrates the healing power of whole foods without added oils in preventing and reversing heart disease. If heart patients adopted this diet, we know that most would not advance their disease and many could actually reverse it.

So, as much as I wish that our government and organizations like the AHA had our best interests at heart, I now know that they do not. As long as lobbyists exist for the dairy, egg, chicken, beef, pork and fish industries, spending huge amounts of money to keep their products on the supermarket shelves, nothing will dramatically change. Their influence over the DGAC will continue to be felt as the truth about the dangers of their products remain hidden from the public. As Americans, we must critically assess any nutrition claim, asking ourselves questions like, "Who funded this study" and "Who sits on these committees that make decisions that can impact my life?" If someone who has worked as part of the animal industry sits on a committee for dietary guidelines, we must insist that this no longer be the case. They most certainly have a vested interest in promoting their product. If guidelines are based on studies conducted by the animal industries, as many are, we must remain skeptical and carefully examine the results. Bias is certainly at play, and the stakes are high. Remember, these guidelines set forth by the DGAC can be deadly.

10

Returning to Chicago

We knew that we would not stay in Texas forever, and after five years we returned to Chicago where my husband had secured another job. We had missed living up north where we could experience all four seasons, each with its own unique beauty. My Texas friends thought I was crazy when I told them I was looking forward to snow! I had always loved cross country skiing and couldn't wait to get back to it. Our relocation did have one downside. It meant my having to close yet another psychotherapy practice, as I contemplated the next move in my professional career.

Nothing really stays the same when you return to a place you have lived in before. Upon our arrival, we stayed in corporate housing while we searched for a home. On my first day out with our realtor, I walked into a house that had the most perfect kitchen for someone like me who loves to cook. I was already thinking about having in-home cooking classes, and this house was just perfect for that! I called Dale and excitedly told him, "I think I've found our house!"

My friends had to get used to a different me from the one I was when we left Chicago five years earlier. The old me loved eating all the foods that my friends ate. Now things were very different. There were some with whom I had remained close and who supported me in my new lifestyle. There were others, however, who did not. I'm not sure why they felt the way they did, but the friendships just didn't continue. I may have changed so much from the person they knew before we left Chicago that we just didn't have that much in common anymore. They were all still eating the animal and dairy products that I had given up, and perhaps they thought of me as being a bit extreme. I knew that I couldn't let their discomfort or disapproval change my mind about the life I had chosen to live. Thankfully, most of my friends were supportive and remain so to this day.

I have learned since early on in this journey that what I am doing sometimes threatens what others believe is a healthy lifestyle choice for themselves. Occasionally a friend will challenge my plant-based regimen, trying to convince me that her animal-based one was the better choice. I don't believe it is productive to preach about eating a WFPD. However, if someone is truly interested in understanding why I live this way, I am happy to tell them. Some are open to exploring it, while others are not. In any case, I remain respectful of an individual's right to make his or her decision.

My own children have had to decide for themselves what choices to make regarding their diets. My two sons continue to eat the standard American diet, while my daughter has made some significant changes in her eating habits, using more plant foods as she plans her meals. For example, when I recently visited her in San Francisco for Thanksgiving, she prepared a plant-based dinner for us that was delicious! Likewise, my son Michael and his wife Heather have been ever so accommodating of our diet, always searching for plant-based recipes that they can prepare for us when we visit them in Ohio. Heather outdoes herself every time. I love her black bean burgers and her sticky sesame cauliflower dish. I also appreciate how my grandchildren bake warm plant-based chocolate chip cookies to enjoy that are sitting on the counter when we arrive. I think had I started eating the way I do now when my kids were young that their eating habits would have been a different story.

I have known individuals who have raised their children from birth with the WFPD and these offspring are thriving. LeAnne Campbell, Executive Director of the Global Roots Project, has raised her two sons eating this way. Both are big and strong young men, now in their 20's, and they have never eaten anything but plants. They are a testament to the benefits of this lifestyle.

There are also stories of how older adults have made the change to a WFPD after a lifetime of eating animal foods. One such person is Gladys Koetsveld, a woman I met in Hawaii in 2015 while attending a week-long program sponsored by Dr. John McDougall. Gladys was well into her 80's and had been suffering from debilitating arthritis. Her daughter had transitioned to the WFPD and started to teach her mother how to do so as well to see if it would alleviate her arthritic symptoms. With very limited mobility and pain, Gladys, unable to enjoy life, decided to give it a try. It was amazing to see the improvement in her health. Within months, she was up and about, no longer needing a cane or walker, and on the Hawaii trip, she joined me snorkeling in the ocean. Meanwhile, her daughter decided to change her career path from a research librarian in Australia to a plant-based nutritionist, working side by side with her partner, Dr. Malcolm Mackey, a physician who practices life style medicine. They have become two of the leading proponents of the WFPD lifestyle through their organization, Plant Based Health Australia.

I have found that one of the most challenging parts of transitioning to a WFPD is learning how to dine at restaurants. What I discovered was that while some chefs try to offer more appealing plant-based dishes, they are often laden with oil, salt and sugar—all ingredients I must avoid for my own health.

What I have found most helpful to do before arriving at a restaurant is to call ahead and ask the chef to please prepare something for me that is healthier. Sometimes these dishes are great but unfortunately often the food is rather bland. It is much easier and better tasting if I just made the food at home. But eating out with friends is a social thing, so I have just accepted the fact that I have to order steamed veggies or a baked potato or salad and call it a day. The point of eating out, after all, is to be with my friends and enjoy the conversation, not to have the best meal of my life.

Having said that, I am hopeful that restaurant chefs across America will start experimenting in their kitchens with some healthful plant-based options. We are well on our way. Chef Del Sroufe, co-owner of The Wellness Forum in Columbus, Ohio, has published many wonderful WFPB cookbooks and travels around the world sharing his love for this way of cooking. He has lost over 200 pounds on the WFPD and is an inspiration to everyone who meets him. Anytime I have the opportunity to talk with a chef or a restaurant owner, I always encourage them to think about offering more oil-free, plant-based options to their customers. I let them know how happy it would make me if they would open restaurants and catering businesses that would fill the niche for no-oil plant-based eaters like myself. The trend for more healthful options, while still in its nascency, is starting to take hold.

In 2017, Plant Pure Café opened its door in Philadelphia, where everything is made without oil! On their menu are rice and bean bowls loaded with veggies, plant wraps, soups and salads. Will stop in when in that area someday.

Dr. Joel Kahn, a cardiologist, launched GreenSpace Café, in Ferndale, Michigan, offering all plant-based healthy options.

In Portland, Oregon, Dale and I discovered a lovely no-oil plant-based café called Herbivoro. The food was delicious! We both ordered the tacos, which were awesome.

Ann Esselstyn and her daughter, Jane Esselstyn, have written a WFPB cookbook, as have LeAnne Campbell, Kim Campbell, Mary McDougall and many others who cook without added oils and very limited sodium. I have recently become acquainted with an artist turned healthcare advocate by the name of Danielle Bussone, who has written a wonderful book called *Time for Change*.[31] Danielle is an excellent cook whose recipes, many of which are flavored with spices, are most enticing.

I have been to various vegan restaurants throughout the United States where the food served is far from healthy. Many of these places use meat "substitutes" made from isolated soy protein. These foods are very popular because they mimic the taste and texture of meat. While it is ok to use them while transitioning to a WFPD, they are not health foods and are not good for our bodies in the long run. Filled with fats, salt and sugar and containing some ingredients that you cannot even pronounce, these foods are best avoided.

The point here is that there is such a thing as an unhealthy plant-based lifestyle. A diet consisting of french fries, potato chips, crackers, cookies and cakes, while plant-based, is certainly not a healthy diet. These foods are laden with fat, salt and sugar. Having a sweet dessert should be a special treat, not daily fare, and using recipes low in fat, salt and sugar are the way to go. What I have found is that by eating lots of whole grains, legumes, fruits and vegetables at every meal, the desire for sweets seems to dissipate. This was my husband's experience. He rarely asks for sweets anymore.

Another challenge faced by those transitioning to a WFPD is how to shop in the grocery store. Reading nutritional labels can be confusing and rather intimidating. I remember my first trip to the grocery store after cleaning out my pantry to start stocking it with plant foods. I spent four hours that day in Whole Foods, reading every label to see what was safe for me to buy and what was not. It was unbelievable to see how many products had oil in them! From breads to soup broths and to many products in between. I quickly learned that the perimeter of the store—where the fruits and vegetables were located—was the place to be. There I would try to purchase organic produce as much as possible because conventional produce is often coated with pesticides and herbicides that are harmful to human health. I choose not to put those into my body anymore. There is a list of foods called The Clean 15 and The Dirty Dozen that can help you decide when to buy organic and when it's ok to go with conventional produce.[32]

The Dirty Dozen tested positive for at least 47 chemicals, with some testing positive for as many as 67. They are:

- Celery
- Peaches
- Strawberries
- Apples
- Domestic blueberries
- Nectarines
- Sweet bell peppers
- Spinach, kale and collard greens
- Cherries
- Imported grapes
- Lettuce

By contrast, the Clean 15 have little to no trace of pesticides. They are:

- Onions
- Avocadoes

- Sweet corn
- Pineapples
- Mango
- Sweet peas
- Asparagus
- Kiwi fruit
- Cabbage
- Eggplant
- Cantaloupe
- Watermelon
- Grapefruit
- Sweet potatoes
- Sweet onions

There are, to be sure, some oil-free products in grocery stores but they are far and few between. A little time spent checking out labels is well worth the effort. What I have found frustrating is that sometimes some formerly oil-free products have been changed to include oil, which I would discover only upon reading the label at home. More reason to check labels even on products that you think are oil-free to make sure that they still are.

In addition, it is important to check sodium levels in foods you purchase. I try to keep my sodium intake to 1500mg per day. In many of the oil-free foods the levels of sodium in their product are quite high. The safest way to avoid getting too much sodium is to eat whole foods and to cook without salt as much as possible. Try experimenting with herbs when seasoning your food. I also use salt substitutes that are rich in potassium (such as Spike seasoning). I think you'll discover a whole new world of taste with the added benefit of lowering your blood pressure naturally.

Please know that I understand that change is difficult. Habits of a lifetime take time to reverse. While my WFPD is now a firmly entrenched part of my lifestyle and the thought of returning to an animal-based diet would never cross my mind, that transition has taken time. Thankfully, I am a pretty good cook (according to Dale and my friends and family), and I'm always interested in trying new recipes. Over the years I have discovered many favorites that are easy to prepare. As my husband has aptly put it, I truly am a "mad scientist" in the kitchen.

Make no mistake, it takes planning and effort to eat this way. Here's some advice I would give to anyone starting out. Choose a day when you can devote several hours to preparing a few meals ahead of time that you can freeze in containers to use as needed. That way you remove the temptation of eating things that are not good for you. Examples of some of the things I freeze are chili, casseroles, pancakes, sauces, sorbets and soups. I've included my favorite recipes for you to try and enjoy in Chapter 19. Just remember to be adventurous in your kitchen and, above all, have fun with it. The foods may be different but they are truly delicious, and I think you will love them as much as I do.

Also know that you can purchase frozen meals from PlantPure Nation. These meals are low in fat, salt and sugar and are oil-free. They are shipped on dry ice directly to your home and are great to have around when you don't have time to put together a meal. They can also be purchased directly at all Albertson grocery stores.

And finally, Engine 2 brand sells oil-free, low fat, low sugar and low sodium products at Whole Foods. Some examples are: cereals, wraps, hummus, pasta sauce, plant milk, and many frozen items including burgers, rice, and stuffed pastas.

11

My Next Chapter

Moving back to Chicago gave me pause to determine what the next chapter of my life would look like. Should I start a new psychotherapy practice for the third time or should I pursue something different? After much thought, it became clear to me that while I still wanted to work as a psychotherapist, I did not want to do it full-time anymore. Instead, I would work part-time in an established group practice and focus the rest of my time and energy on helping individuals transition to a WFPD.

In preparation for this shift in my career focus, I enrolled in the plant-based certificate program at eCornell University and The T. Colin Campbell Center for Nutrition Studies. This six-week certification program further educated me about the science behind the WFPD, which in turn I was able to impart to others in a variety of ways. I had first heard about this program when Dale and I went on an all-vegan Caribbean cruise vacation, sponsored by Holistic Holidays at Sea. It was at that time that I heard Dr. T. Colin Campbell speak about his work concerning the link between cancer and nutrition. I had already read his book, *The China Study*, and was in awe of this man who had devoted his entire professional life to the study of diet and disease. His course featured numerous guest lecturers, including Dr. Caldwell Esselstyn, Dr. Douglas Lisle, and many others, who tackled subjects like heart disease, diabetes, autoimmune diseases, cancer and the effects of animal farming on the environment.

Students in the program included doctors, nurses, nurse practitioners, physician's assistants, nutrititionists, dieticians, and other healthcare professionals and lay people like myself. We listened to online lectures, wrote papers, and took tests in order to receive our certificates. There were also online discussions led by instructors that gave us the opportunity to discuss what we had learned and ask for any needed clarification of the course material. Being all science-based, this program was not an easy one to complete, especially for someone like me who did not have a science background. However, by the end of the six weeks, and after much hard work, I received my certificate, feeling much better informed about the benefits of the WFPD.

That Holistic Holiday at Seas cruise we had taken had 1,500 plant-based passengers on board, requiring two large dining rooms to accommodate all of us. One of those dining rooms served food devoid of any oil. What a pleasure it was to be served all week long with those who ate the way we did. During the day, I attended health-related lectures, exercised, went on excursions and just plain relaxed. We met some lovely people on this trip, some of whom we still keep in touch with today. But most importantly, we knew that we were not alone on this journey.

I was fortunate to have participated in a panel discussion during the cruise that focused on recovery from life-threatening illnesses. I was able to tell my story about my near fatal heart attack and surgery and what I was doing to prevent this from ever happening to me again. Others on the panel had similar life-altering events, including bouts with cancer, diabetes, and autoimmune diseases. It was fascinating to hear their stories and to see how all of us had healed our bodies through a WFPD.

The question for me after completing the certificate program in plant-based nutrition was, "So what am I going to do with all of this newfound knowledge?" It had always been my intention to start a cooking class and to teach about the prevention and reversal of heart disease. I got busy doing both upon my return to Chicago. I contacted an adult education program in the area where I lived and submitted a proposal to teach "How To Heart Attack Proof Yourself With a Whole Foods No-oil Plant-based Diet." My proposal was accepted and my first class was scheduled. We had about ten people register for that class. Based on the research of Dr. Caldwell Esselstyn, author of *Prevent and Reverse Heart Disease,* I prepared an informative PowerPoint presentation with the help of my tech-savvy husband. I also prepared a buffet of delicious no-oil plant-based foods that we ate together after my lecture.

We had a very special treat during that first class. Dr. Esselstyn kindly agreed to phone into the class after my presentation to say a few words to the attendees and to answer any questions. I'll never forget the look on my students' faces when they knew they were getting direct access to this doctor who had done the research we had just talked about! Dr. Esselstyn was so kind and generous with his time. As I mentioned earlier, we had first spoken on the phone after he had watched my interview on *Women Who Lead.* He and his wife Ann have since made themselves available to me whenever I have had any questions or needed advice. This is the kind of doctor who makes a real difference in people's lives. His dedication to ending heart disease is unrelenting. He has made, and will continue to make, a priceless difference in people's lives by saving them from the ravages of heart disease.

Class participants who tasted my food, consisting of butternut squash soup, lentil joes (a recipe from Ann Esselstyn), banana bread, fruit smoothies and a chick pea salad, were pleasantly surprised by how delicious it was. My students were encouraged to bring storage containers to class so that they could take home any leftovers to share with their family and friends. And that's how it all started.

I have since taught this class on many more occasions, helping to change the way people eat, one person at a time. And my success rate has been pretty good! I'd guess that about half of each class started to transition to this way of eating, and many have maintained their new lifestyle. Comments on the course evaluations included, "Life-saving information," "I'm sold," and "Sherry has inspired me to live a healthy life from this day on." There is nothing more rewarding to me than helping people make this change because I know it can only mean good things for their health for the rest of their lives.

In addition to my class on the prevention and reversal of heart disease, I wanted to teach people how to cook plant foods without added oil. So I developed a cooking class by creating my very own Meetup group called "Lincolnshire Vegan No-oil Cooking Classes." Anyone living within driving distance of my home can join the group for free by signing up at my site. I charge only $20 per class, which seems very reasonable, considering that participants create a full course meal that they enjoy once prepared.

We now have over 300 members, and the group keeps on growing. Of course, I cannot have all of them in my home at one time, but I am able to accommodate up to 18 individuals. What is nice about each class is that we have some regular attendees as well as newcomers. After class, I post the recipes on my site for all members to enjoy.

Each month we decide on a theme for recipes that are relatively simple to make. Some of those include Asian, Mediterranean, Italian and Mexican cooking. We also have prepared soups, casseroles, sauces, appetizers and desserts.

Helping me come up with all of these ideas is my friend Karen Kornick, co-coordinator of our group. Karen is a registered nurse who teaches health in a suburban middle school. Her students are very lucky to have her as their teacher as she has introduced them to plant-based nutrition as part of her curriculum.

That approach has, however, met with some resistance. Karen actually was called down to the principal's office for having spoken of the deleterious effects of dairy products, which had led one student to inform his mother that he was going to refrain from drinking milk forever. This did not sit well with her, who felt it was audacious on Karen's part to suggest that dairy carried harmful health effects. To her credit, Karen remains undeterred in educating her students about the benefits of a WFPD. She even went so far as to show the film *What The Health* to her class, which led to much discussion among her students.

So, you might be wondering how in the world do I teach 18 people every month how to cook oil-free plant-based meals. Here's what I do. When students arrive, they are assigned to a cooking station. At that station are all of the ingredients and cooking tools they need to create their recipe. They then work together in groups of four. When each group completes their dish we all sit together in my kitchen to talk about the recipes and then enjoy the meal together. I always throw in some education about the benefits of a WFPD to reinforce why we are eating this way in the first place. We then end our evening by opening the floor for discussion and questions. It is always a very lively, informative and fun event.

This cooking class format is working beautifully. It has become clear to me that no matter how much information we learn about why we should eat a WFPD, it is not until you actually prepare and taste the food that you see how marvelous it really is. That's what ultimately sells people on the idea that they can transition to this way of living. And the bonus of course for all of my students is that they are improving their health just by changing what they eat for breakfast, lunch and dinner.

I have also incorporated my very own 21 Day Challenge for members of my cooking classes who are desirous of making a clean transition to the WFPD. Each is advised to make his or her physician aware of this dietary change (this is especially important for those with Type 2 diabetes, who may need to lower their medications over the course of the 21 Day Challenge). They are also instructed to have their cholesterol, blood pressure and glucose levels checked prior to and at the completion of the Challenge. During this three-week period, I provide individual coaching through weekly phone calls, during which I review menus, offer suggestions, provide support, and discuss how to handle difficult situations such as eating at restaurants or eating at a friend's home. One woman, suffering from an arthritic condition and high cholesterol, saw her overall cholesterol level drop by over 50 points at the end of the Challenge, and her LDL cholesterol significantly improved. She also reported having more energy, but, most importantly, she experienced a significant reduction in her joint pain—all this in just 21 days!

12

Making A Difference

I am a firm believer that we can all make a difference in this world no matter how big or small our contribution. Having almost died from heart disease, I have made educating others on how to avoid this fate a top priority. The way I have chosen to do this is by teaching courses on heart attack prevention and reversal and conducting no-oil plant-based cooking classes.

What I want my readers to know, however, is that I cannot do this alone. As the African proverb teaches, "If you want to travel fast, go alone. If you want to travel far, go together." It will surely take a village to bring about change in the way Americans eat. So, to collaborate on how to bring about such changes, Dale and I decided to attend the first Global Roots Total Health Experience in the Dominican Republic. This conference was presented by Dr. LeAnne Campbell, Executive Director of The Global Roots project. There, the 60 people in attendance listened to informative lectures on the most current scientific evidence on the WFPD as well as participated in discussions about ways to impart this information to individuals in our respective communities.

Speakers at the conference included Dr. T. Colin Campbell (nutritional biochemist and author of *The China Study* and of over 300 research papers on cancer and nutrition), Dr. Michael C. Hollie (member of the American College of Lifestyle Medicine and founder of Dinner with the Doctor program in Chattanooga, Tennessee), Dr. John Kelly (an Irish doctor who wrote *Stop Feeding Your Cancer*), Dr. Amy J. Lanou (University of North Carolina professor and senior nutrition scientist for the Physicians Committee for Responsible Medicine), and Ms. Michelle Burton, MBA (community activist from Los Angeles, California and fundraising head for AltaMed, the nation's largest community health center).

Together we brainstormed regarding different strategies we might use to effect change in how we look at nutrition and disease prevention. We asked ourselves, "Was it better to work at the establishment level within the government or health organizations or was a grass roots movement the most efficacious way to bring about change?"

Some thought that teaching medical students the science behind the WFPD was an essential first step in educating new doctors about the health benefits of eating this way. At present, most medical students receive very little or no training in plant-based nutrition. Fortunately, this is slowly starting to change as physicians like John McDougall and others are teaching these courses in medical schools across the United States. I myself recently had the opportunity to give an interview, sponsored by the Physicians Committee for Responsible Medicine, about the importance of this medical training in a movie to be viewed by medical students.

Undoubtedly, this exposure to the science behind this diet as a means to prevent and even reverse chronic illnesses marks a very important change that will certainly influence their treatment of patients. Hopefully this will lead more and more doctors to retire their prescription pads in favor of an approach to treatment in which plant-based nutrition figures prominently.

At the conference we also learned that medical symposiums across the country were now offering physicians the opportunity to gain more knowledge about plant-based nutrition and its benefits. One example of this was a recent meeting of the American College of Cardiology at which the then president, Dr. Kim Williams, presented information to his fellow cardiologists on using plant-based nutrition to treat heart disease. This was a big step toward educating doctors working in the field of cardiology.

Another topic that we discussed at the conference dealt with how we could work effectively through governmental channels to drive change. Dr. T. Colin Campbell shared with us his experiences in doing this while serving on governmental committees. Unfortunately, his efforts to inform the public about the health risks associated with eating animal-based foods were met with fierce resistance at every level, especially by the lobbyist groups who had a vested interest in keeping their animal products on the shelves of American grocery stores. These groups also continue to proclaim that their products are good for us and should form part of a balanced diet.

Here are some examples of how these industries continue to fool the American public.

- For decades, the dairy industry has been promoting its products as health-promoting. They tell us that milk makes our bones strong. What they never tell you is that the scientific literature does not support that notion and, in fact, has shown that when we ingest animal products (including milk), the calcium in our bones is leached out to neutralize the highly acidic environment in our bodies that comes from eating animal foods. In short, bones are weakened, leading to the development of osteoporosis and fractures.[33]

- Milk is also responsible for introducing one of the most harmful carcinogens into our system in the form of casein, the protein component of milk. It is also implicated in the development of Type I diabetes, a life-long disease with devastating consequences. The cholesterol in dairy products also contributes to the development of heart disease because of its high amount of saturated fat. Yet, claims that milk is an essential part of a healthy diet remain firmly entrenched in the thinking of many who know nothing about the deleterious effects of dairy products. Do you know of any other species that drinks the milk of another species? There is a reason why this never occurs. Cow's milk is the perfect food for growing baby calves, but it was never intended to be the perfect food for humans. The United States, a country with one of the highest rates of dairy consumption, also has the dubious distinction of having one of the highest rates of risk for bone fractures and osteoporosis.[34]

- Remember when Oprah Winfrey was sued by the cattle industry for even suggesting that meat was not good for our health? And that was Oprah Winfrey! As Dr. Campbell expressed during the Global Roots Conference, he has given up on the idea that the way to get the truth out about nutrition is to work through governmental agencies. It just won't happen that way. Consider this. The United States Department of Agriculture, through its Dietary Guidelines Committee, is responsible for establishing dietary guidelines by advising Americans on the components of a healthy diet.

- However, as a lawsuit brought by The Physicians Committee for Responsible Medicine (PCRM) in the 1990s revealed, the Dietary Guidelines Committee included nine members with ties to the very industries whose foods were promoted in the guidelines! This manifest conflict of interest has no place in policymaking that has such serious effects on the health of all Americans. We deserve better from our government.

As we continued our discussion on this topic, some suggested that we move the Dietary Guidelines Committee from the auspices of the Department of Agriculture into a neutral body situated elsewhere in the government. I think this is an excellent idea. No one associated with any food industry should be serving on a committee that makes recommendations to the American public about what we should be eating for our optimal health.

One other idea that came out of the Global Roots Conference, and one with the most potential to change how Americans eat, is for informed citizens to start grass roots movements with the objective of spreading the word in their local communities about the health benefits of eating a WFPD. This is what I am doing through my classes as are others throughout the world.

We live in a country of free enterprise. I believe we should give people information supported by scientific evidence that will allow them to make informed decisions about their diet and then let the free market decide in which direction to proceed. I realize what a monumental paradigm shift it would be for farmers to transition from raising animals for human consumption to growing produce instead. But just think about what a wonderful world it would be if this actually happened. People would be well and our humongous health care costs would once and for all be contained! And better yet, we could then use the grains once fed to animals to provide food for all the people in the world so that no human would ever have to die of starvation again. And just as importantly, our environment would no longer be degraded by the practices associated with raising animals for human consumption. No more deforestation, wasting of water or release of harmful gases into our atmosphere from animal farming. I want to be a part of that world.

And all of this is starting to happen. More and more dairy companies are moving away from selling cow's milk to transitioning to plant-based milks. Companies producing plant foods, from nut cheeses to burgers that taste like beef, are popping up everywhere. I personally am unable to eat these foods as they contain oil, salt and sugars. However, it certainly is a sign that the food industry is responding to the demand for more plant-based choices.

Thinking about what animals must endure as they go to slaughter has given me a new perspective on suffering and how we must avoid hurting other living beings. I would never think of killing my pet cat or dog in order to eat them, so what makes the life of a chicken, pig, lamb, rabbit or cow any less worthy? When I think about the lack of quality of their lives in order that humans can feast on their flesh, I feel sickened and saddened. Have you ever wondered what it would be like to be kept in a small, contained area, surrounded by others in your species, living in filthy conditions only to be led off to be butchered? Animals feel pain. They even feel anxiety and know fear. Make no mistake about it. I believe in a much kinder and gentler world where we do not cause pain and suffering to any living being. One can only hope that our world will move in that direction, one where all living things are honored and valued.

So it's at this grassroots level of advocacy for the truth about the American diet where I am at today. Nelson Campbell, son of Dr. T. Colin Campbell, has started such a movement, appropriately named PlantPure Nation. As I mentioned earlier, there is a documentary by that name that explores the state of our health and government's reluctance to encourage citizens to embrace a whole foods plant-based life, largely because of the resistance they have encountered from the animal and dairy industries. To that end, Campbell has started a nationwide movement of local "pods," i.e., groups, to help promote this movement.

The good news is, all across America, change is happening. People are meeting in homes, community centers, churches, and schools, working together to change the way Americans eat. However, it will take the collaborative efforts of many people to bring about these changes. You too can help. Start with yourself. Invite friends and family over for a meal and let them experience the goodness of eating this way. Take courses. Hold cooking classes as I do or teach in your community. Start a book club where you read everything out there about plant-based nutrition. Take fresh fruits and vegetables to schools. Lobby our school systems to go plant-based for the future of our children's health. Encourage chefs across America to use their talents to create plant-based dishes that will be served in their restaurants and catering businesses. Every little bit helps and it is with these efforts that our numbers will multiply.

And multiple we have. Veganism has grown 500% since 2014 in the United States: as of 2017, 6% of Americans identify as vegan—up from only 1% three years earlier, according to a report by Global Data Research entitled *Top Trends in Prepared Foods in 2017*.[35]

One of the most effective ways to improve the health of Americans would be for insurance companies to compensate physicians who educate their patients about plant-based nutrition as a means to prevent or reverse heart disease, diabetes, autoimmune diseases, and even some forms of cancer. Medicare is already onboard in this effort. We must reward our doctors who take the time to teach their patients about these lifesaving changes. Blood work results don't lie. Blood pressure readings don't lie. Glucose levels don't lie. Permanent reductions in all of these health metrics as a result of eating this way should incentivize insurance companies to appropriately compensate physicians.

I understand that doctors work very hard to earn their medical degrees. I certainly don't blame them for what they were taught at the time they attended medical school. But the world is changing, and we now need them to have a new focus—one centered on wellness by using whole foods to treat our chronic diseases. This will allow doctors to move away from simply treating symptoms with medications and procedures in favor of getting at the root causes of illness. Give plants a chance! No side effects, just health.

There will always be some doctors who resist recommending a plant-based regimen, but we must make them accountable for providing us what science is telling us is best for us. Particularly given the fact that withholding such information could lead to loss of life. I remember seeing a blood specialist in Houston after my heart attack and bypass surgery who told me that he wouldn't waste his time telling people to eat plant-based because they would never listen to him anyway. This was a doctor who was very overweight and clearly not in the best of health himself. If you look at what Dr. Esselstyn has accomplished with the most critically ill heart patients at the Cleveland Clinic through counseling about plant-based nutrition, the benefits are clear. The public wants and deserves the truth and can make up their own mind about what to do with the information. I have complete faith in people that they will make better choices when given this knowledge.

I think there are distinct parallels between our efforts to educate people about the perils of the standard American diet and the dangers of smoking. To be sure, it took many years for doctors to inform their patients about the clear health risks that attend smoking. It was only when faced with the incontrovertible evidence of the lethal effects of tobacco that physicians began to apprise their patients of them. Likewise, while it will no doubt take time for the medical community as a whole to recognize the dangers of animal-based foods, we must be unrelenting in our efforts to effect a similar change in terms of what they advise their patients. If I were a cardiologist, I would derive tremendous satisfaction knowing I had something to offer my patients that could truly save their lives.

I often think about Dr. Esselstyn's response to the question, "Isn't changing your diet like this extreme and rather radical?" His reply was something to the effect that isn't it extreme to cut open someone's chest and take a vein from another part of their body to create a new arterial pathway bypassing the blocked coronary artery? Of course it is. Not to mention the aftereffects of such a radical surgery. For me, it included some cognitive difficulties with memory, loss of time from work (4 months), physical weakness, and a depression that took months to come out of. And all of this could have been avoided had I only known what I know now.

13

My Search for A Plant-Based Doctor

My own experience in trying to find doctors who understand why I am eating a WFPD has been very challenging to say the least. Returning to Chicago after a five-year absence, I visited with my former internist to re-establish myself as her patient. She was caring and attentive and we had a wonderful rapport. However, I quickly realized that we were not on the same page when it came to disease prevention. Her first line of defense relied on drugs to treat symptoms. She was so firmly rooted in her beliefs that she became upset with me when she learned that my cardiologist had decided to take me off of my blood pressure medications because my pressure was extremely low. He wanted to see how I would fare without them and, if not needed, to discontinue them permanently. She made it clear that she did not favor this approach because of my family history of high blood pressure and heart disease. Furthermore, she insinuated that I would need medications for life. She completely ruled out the possibility that lifestyle changes could trump any genetic predisposition I might have towards high blood pressure. Rather than debate her on this subject, I decided to look for another doctor who was more aligned with my thinking and who was open to trying whole foods first as a way to prevent disease.

I finally found a doctor who was a vegan. She was very young and fresh out of her residency. What I learned from her was that she did eat a mainly plant-based diet but still used olive oil, which she thought was essential for optimal health. Once again, I was confronted with a physician who, while subscribing to a diet much like mine, was not adequately trained in nutrition to know that olive oil was artery-clogging and nitric oxide-inhibiting and thus impeded optimal endothelial cell functioning. She was plainly misinformed, presumably because she had not been educated about the benefits of a WFPD. She remained a primary care physician for only a few years, having decided to pursue a position in an acute care center instead.

The first cardiologist I saw when I returned to Illinois was a plant-based cardiologist in Kenosha, Wisconsin by the name of Kevin Fullin. He had practiced traditional cardiology for years until he had knee replacement surgery. While recuperating at home, he happened to watch the documentary *Forks Over Knives*. Watching it led him to sign up to take the Certificate Program in Plant-based Nutrition (the very program that I had taken), as well as a program with Dr. John McDougall in Santa Rosa, California, in an effort to become more informed about the prevention and reversal of heart disease through plant-based nutrition.

Once certified in plant-based nutrition, he started a prevention and reversal program of his own. Upon entering his office, the first thing one sees is a television showing *Forks Over Knives*. It was so wonderful to see it playing.

All of my cardiac follow-up visits have shown great results. My heart is doing fine, and during my last stress test, I shocked the technician when I started running quite vigorously on the treadmill until the test was concluded. She told me she had never seen anyone with my history of heart disease put on such a good performance on the treadmill. Thanks to the power of plants!

My cholesterol at that time ran close to 105 and my blood pressure was normal. I did not require any heart medications except for a very small dose of Crestor (5 mg) along with a baby aspirin and Vitamin B12 (necessary if you eat plant-based). The great news for those who can come off of medications is that plants don't have side effects. Unfortunately, prescription medications usually do, and if you listen to the commercials on television, you quickly learn what they are and what harm they can bring, including death.

Fast forward to 2017. Since then, I am seeing another plant-based cardiologist, Dr. Kim Williams. He was serving as the President of the American College of Cardiology when I met him in 2016. Dr. Williams transitioned to this way of eating many years ago and is a shining example of a doctor who practices what he preaches. He is a true inspiration for his colleagues and patients alike.

Dr. Williams and I work together to ensure my continued good health. He knows how disciplined I am when it comes to my plant-based diet so it was difficult for me to accept his recommendation that I needed to resume taking blood pressure medication. For whatever reason, no matter how well I eat, it remains higher than Dr. Williams and I are comfortable with. Having to take drugs is not something I am happy about, but I recognize that it is necessary in my case. The bottom line is that I want to stay alive well into old age, and if it means having to take some medications, I am on board. As Dr. Williams put it, "You are doing so well and need so little medication BECAUSE of your diet. It is just that for some people, diet alone won't reduce your blood pressure or cholesterol enough." What's important is that we partner with physicians who let us try using only food as medicine FIRST! If and when we need more, it is important to be open to that and to embrace what modern medicine has to offer.

I am now seeing Dr. Marcy Kamen as my internist. While

we are not exactly the same when it comes to our diets, she following more of the Mediterranean diet, she is respectful of mine and listens to me, and most importantly, we team together to promote my best health. An example of this has to do with what some might call a low Vitamin D level. She wanted me to take a Vitamin D supplement but was open to my trying to get direct sunlight during the summer months to raise the levels naturally. I appreciated her willingness to respect my wish to avoid taking supplements unless there was a pressing need for them. She also graciously accepted an article I brought to her written by Dr. John McDougall on the subject of Vitamin D, which discussed reasons why he does not prescribe this supplement to his patients.[36] Dr. Kamen is a good example of working with a physician who, while not totally plant-based, is nevertheless open to learning new things.

For those of you looking to find a plant-based physician, I would suggest you refer to https://VegDocs.com. Another resource is the American College of Lifestyle Medicine at https://lifestylemedicine.org.

If you are fortunate enough to live in or near one of the following areas, you will find some of the best plant-based physicians, as follows:

- Washington D.C.: Dr. Neal Barnard
- Santa Rosa, California: Dr. John McDougall
- Rochester, New York: Dr. Thomas Campbell
- Portland, Oregon: Dr. Craig McDougall
- Houston, Texas: Dr. Baxter Montgomery
- Detroit, Michigan: Dr. Joel Kahn
- Chicago, Illinois: Dr. Kim Williams
- Cleveland, Ohio: Dr. Caldwell Esselstyn
- San Francisco, California: Dr. Dean Ornish

- Los Angeles, California: Dr. Alone Pulde and Dr. Matthew Lederman

As Dr. Baxter Montgomery aptly put it:

American medicine needs to change its focus. Medical practice has become a process of prescribing medicines and procedures to treat the side effects of the bad foods we eat. The key issue for true health is a healthy lifestyle, and the core of that lifestyle is optimal nutrition. That needs to be the focus of our practice.[37]

These are just a few of the talented and dedicated physicians who are making a true difference in the lives of their patients by using food as first resort in preventing and reversing chronic and life-threatening diseases. In coming years, I expect to see our choices expand as more and more doctors pursue this professional path.

14

The Mind-Body Connection for Healing

As a practicing psychotherapist and life coach, I felt it was important for me to devote a chapter to the healing powers of yoga, qi gong (a meditation in motion), and meditation. I started my mindfulness journey many years ago by practicing yoga with my beloved friend and teacher, Ceily Levy. Here is what I have learned.

For many of us, life is exceedingly busy. We have our work, our families, our friends and our special interests, to all of which we try our best to give our full attention. Sleep for many has become a luxury rather than a necessity, leading to a nation of sleep-deprived individuals. Taking time to slow down and recharge our energy has unfortunately not been a priority for many of us.

Ceily taught me how to be in the present moment and that by doing so I am giving myself one of life's most valuable gifts. So, what does this mean? Consider how our minds work. We are constantly thinking about what happened yesterday, what's on our to do list for today, and what tomorrow will bring. Our minds chatter away in a relentless review all day long. Learning to quiet the mind is something that requires effort. Because doing so does not come naturally or easily to most of us, having

patience and showing kindness to self throughout the process
are key. Practicing yoga, qi gong and meditation are ways to
slow things down and appreciate every single moment of life.
It made me realize that all I really have is this moment. And
most importantly, it taught me how to show gratitude for the
precious nature of my life.

My practices also informed me to let go of thoughts that
were not serving me well. There are situations in life that
are not healthy for us, and to be able to accept and move on
without reviewing these life situations continuously is another
gift we can give to ourselves. So, when I see myself focusing on a
negative situation, I immediately attend to my breath and allow
the thought to pass by like a cloud in the sky. How liberating it
has become for me to do so.

I work with people in my psychotherapy practice who come
to me with tremendous worry and anxiety. Rather than sending
them off to a psychiatrist for psychotropic medications, I will
first suggest mindfulness practices as ways of quieting the
mind (along with talking to me in counseling). When I hear
back from them after they have started to incorporate these
practices into their daily lives, I often learn how amazed they
feel once able to attain a state of stillness and to find their once
racing minds slowly quieting down. This letting go allows for a
free flow of energy that enables us to live life to the fullest.

We are all pushed to the edge at times, when everything
just seems to stop and the fears, worries and anxieties seem
to overtake us. Imagine having the skill to breathe and come
back to the present moment, with a resolve to be still and
release the feelings that are so troublesome to us. Yoga, qi
gong, and meditation are powerful tools for everyone to have
at their disposal.

I am reminded of a study at The University of Wisconsin
where soldiers with severe post-traumatic stress disorder (PTSD)
were instructed on the use of meditation to see if their PTSD

symptoms could be reduced.[38] Those suffering from PTSD often have flashbacks of the traumatic events they have witnessed or participated in, suffer from anxiety and depression and are often quite agitated. Soldiers were interviewed throughout the study to measure their PTSD symptoms and were given a brain wave scan to monitor the activity in their brains. What the study found was that after practicing meditation, the soldiers all experienced a reduction in their PTSD symptoms, and their brain scans showed a gradual reduction of their brain wave activity. Soldiers also reported an ability to use their breathing as a tool to calm themselves when they would start to experience any anxiety symptoms. In many cases, meditation practices could replace or reduce medications for the reduction of anxiety.

Children can also benefit from practicing yoga. In "Just Breathe: A Documentary on Kids and Mindfulness," we are witness to children practicing yoga and meditation as they learn how to calm themselves when feeling angry, stressed or anxious. I am reminded of one little boy in the film who struggled with anger and anxiety. He would often lash out at classmates, causing disruption to the classroom. He also had fears that were interfering with the enjoyment of his life. Through the practice of yoga, he was able to calm himself and face his fears with the loving support of his teachers. He also learned how to breathe mindfully when the anger within would rise up, resulting in him having better relationships with his classmates. The power of yoga to heal is very real and is something valuable to be taught to all children.

For me personally, after my near-death experience, I knew that changing my diet was my first order of business. However, my next priority was changing my frame of mind. I wanted to rid myself of any unnecessary tension and conflict and surround myself with people who were good for me.

I learned that I was not the glue that had to hold relationships together anymore. I wanted people in my life who brought me joy and who loved me unconditionally. This meant having to let go of some who were doing just the opposite. It was a painful process at first, but as I write today, I have a life that is full of joy, compassion, love and true friendships with those that surround me.

Practicing yoga, qi gong and meditation have helped me in a way for which I will be forever grateful. I usually practice in the morning. Afterwards I go to work where I will be sitting for the rest of the day counseling others. I have often heard from my clients that they feel a calmness and peacefulness while in my presence. My hope is that they will learn how to cultivate the same feeling in their own lives as they navigate through whatever challenges they might face.

For those of us with heart disease, it is a reminder to reevaluate our relationships and to make those changes that will serve us well for the rest of our lives. Our diet is very important, but our mental state is just as vital as we heal from our disease.

15

Finding My Voice: Challenging the Medical Establishment

To advocate for what you believe in means to stand up and let your voice be heard. As you have learned in previous chapters, I have had to speak up on numerous occasions to advocate for what I believe are the most health-promoting choices regarding heart disease. It would be very easy to just give up and say to myself, "This is too hard," or "I don't like it when others don't like what I have to say," but somehow, I persevere. It is too important to throw one's hands up in frustration and simply give up. The work to educate the public about the WFPD is on the shoulders of all of us.

While living in Cleveland many years ago, I regularly read a local publication that frequently featured health articles written by prominent physicians from The Cleveland Clinic and University Hospitals of Cleveland. Often, they would give dietary advice.

Some of the offered advice was so blatantly at variance with what I have learned about optimal health that I felt compelled to write to the editor to express my concern and to present a different solution to the problems they addressed. I was like a pesky little bug that would just not go away, but to the editor's credit, he published every one of my responses in the letters to the editorial section of the newspaper.

I will never know how many people read my responses and paid attention to them, but at least I know I am not a silent observer who will let these less than optimal pieces of nutritional advice from physicians go unanswered.

Here is a sampling of some of the advice given by these doctors and a few of my rejoinders.

Posted: Wednesday, May 8, 2013 5:15 pm

Set sail for a Mediterranean diet

Dr. Roy Buchinsky

Cleveland Jewish News

No need to cruise the Aegean Sea to reap the benefits of a heart-healthy Mediterranean diet. Your body can enjoy the rewards of this first-rate diet right here in Cleveland. If you stock your refrigerator and pantry correctly, you can leisurely dine with friends and loved ones on meals of fresh fish, seasonal fruit and vegetables, platters of green and black olives accompanied by crusty whole-grain bread dipped in olive oil, and a side of whole wheat pasta. Add a glass of red wine and, to quote Ira Gershwin, "who can ask for anything more?"

The truth is, this healthy, natural eating style is pleasing to the taste buds and proven to help maintain a vital, robust body. Research has shown that a traditional Mediterranean diet, characterized by a high intake of fruits, vegetables, whole grains, nuts, beans, olive oil; a moderate intake of fish and red wine; and low intake of dairy products and red meat, provides oodles of micronutrients, antioxidants, vitamins and minerals. It also reduces the risk of stroke, heart attack and heart-related diseases by as much as 30 percent.

If that is not enough to make you say bye-bye to slabs of Aunt Bertha's brisket, a Mediterranean diet also reduces cancer and cancer mortality, Parkinson's and Alzheimer's disease, obesity and type 2 diabetes.

If this Mediterranean diet is still Greek to you, imagine a four-tiered food pyramid, a concept popularized by Oldways, a nonprofit food and nutrition education association that looks to the past for guidance. On this pyramid the most important tier is the bottom, which includes fruits, vegetables, grains (mostly whole), olive oil, beans, nuts, legumes, seeds, herbs and spices. You should base every meal on these foods. The next tier is fish and seafood – to eat often, at least twice a week. The next tier calls for moderate amounts of poultry, eggs, cheese and yogurt. And if you really want to stay in fighting form and help colonize Mars, skip red meats and sugary sweets.

The beauty of a Mediterranean diet is that it can be enjoyed all year long – including the upcoming dairy-rich holiday of Shavuot. You can celebrate the giving of the Torah to the Jews on Mount Sinai without consuming a platter of pan-fried cheese blintzes and a hearty slice of cheesecake topped with sweetened whipped cream. You can still enjoy your blintzes and the holiday too by using low-fat ricotta cheese, Greek yogurt or tofu in your dairy dishes; add some seasonal fruit and the harvest holiday will reap good-tasting, healthy benefits.

Mediterranean diet tips

- Go nuts – enjoy a handful of dry roasted peanuts, almonds, walnuts, pistachios and cashews. Avoid honey roasted or seasoned nuts cooked in oil and read peanut butter labels carefully to ensure no nasty hydrogenated fats or salt has been added.
- Oil spills – replace artery-clogging butter with healthy fats like extra-virgin olive oil and canola oil
- Spice up your life - use herbs and spices rather than salt to flavor foods
- Get hooked on fish – enjoy salmon, mackerel, herring, lake trout, sardines and albacore tuna, which are high in omega-3 fatty acids
- Fruits and veggies – produce will produce a healthier you
- Holy cow – choose low-fat milk, cheese and yogurt
- L'Chaim– enjoy a glass of red wine – the daily wine recommendations are 5 ounces for women and 10 ounces for

men. Purple grape juice can also do the trick.

- Move it – daily exercise of 30-60 minutes is important and a regular workout even includes pushing your chair away from the dinner table

Are you ready to cruise the Mediterranean with me?

Here's my response to Dr. Buchinsky:

Posted: Wednesday, May 22, 2013 10:45 am

Mediterranean diet facts off target

Heart disease is the No. 1 killer of men and women in the United States, affecting 36 percent of Americans, but it is preventable by eating an oil-free, whole foods, plant-based diet. Dr. Roy Buchinsky believes that a 30 percent risk reduction for heart disease by consuming the Mediterranean diet is impressive and he advocates this lifestyle in his article. ("Set sail for a Mediterranean diet without leaving home," May 10)

However, the Lyon Diet Heart Study found that 25 percent of those cardiac patients in the experimental group who ate the Mediterranean diet either had another significant cardiac event or had died after four years. These are horrific results for a non-malignant disease.

Dr. Caldwell Esselstyn's study of 17 seriously ill heart patients at the Cleveland Clinic who adhered to a whole foods, plant-based diet had no further cardiac events after 12 years, and some had a reversal of their heart disease. You can read about this study in his book, *Prevent And Reverse Heart Disease*.

Americans deserve the truth about how to prevent and reverse heart disease. In promoting the Mediterranean diet as a means to achieving this goal, Buchinsky does your readers a significant disservice.

Sherry Shrallow

Houston

Posted: Thursday, October 8, 2015 12:10 pm

Beetroot, borscht to the rescue

Dr. Michael Roizen

Special to the CJN

According to the best current science, beetroot juice, aka beet juice, and by inference, borscht, a major product of beetroots, may be a food that fosters energy to make you feel years younger by changing the amount of nitric oxide your arteries produce. According to several studies, even borscht made with veggie stock and beets prepared in olive oil, and no meat products or foods with saturated fat added in, probably fits.

Is beet juice, or borscht properly prepared, a super food? Yes, because, according to studies on its effect on animals, beet juice restores arterial function and increases exercise capacity and stamina in all ages. Ingesting it increases nitric oxide synthesis in the cells lining your arteries.

That nitric oxide is a gas that dilates your artery system, allowing greater blood flow and nutrients in and out of your tissues. It is the substance that dilates the heart when people use nitroglycerin, and it dilates the arteries to sexual organs in both men and women, enabling better erections and lubrication; it even dilates the urethra, allowing fewer symptoms of benign prostatic hypertrophy, or prostate gland enlargement.

The one worry I have about beet juice is that it may raise your blood sugar too quickly. While they have a relatively high glycemic index, beets are relatively low in carbohydrate load so the glycemic load (the real chance your blood sugar will spike) is relatively low. Nevertheless, you can take sips over the entire day of your three pints, or drink a pint 30 minutes after ingesting 70 grams of healthy fat (as in six walnut halves or a little bit of olive oil). Remember to decrease calories in the rest of your diet if you choose to try this super food.

More data have accumulated, which have reaffirmed that substituting saturated fat with a healthy fat like olive oil or with nuts (walnuts, mainly, along with almonds and hazelnuts) decreased breast cancer over 60 percent, heart disease and stroke 30 percent. Further data, derived from a database of 133,000 people, affirms that saturated fat, compared to other fats, increased heart disease risk by 25 percent.

Here are this month's action steps:

- See if you like beet juice. Try a pint three times a day for a week and see if you have more energy (cut out another dish with an equal amount of calories when you add the beet juice)
- Try to make some healthful borscht.

Dr. Michael Roizen writes about wellness for the Cleveland Jewish News. He is chief wellness officer and chair of the Wellness Institute at Cleveland Clinic. Follow him on Twitter @YoungDrMike.

Here's my reply to Dr. Roizen:

Posted: Thursday, November 5, 2015 11:00 am

Roizen misses the mark

Regarding Dr. Michael Roizen's article, ("Beetroot, borscht to the rescue," Oct. 9) he is to be commended for extolling the virtues of beets as part of a healthy diet. Unfortunately, the article misses the mark in a number of other respects.

More specifically, his recommendation to use olive oil, as well as his characterization of it as a healthy fat, is wholly at odds with current scientific literature regarding heart disease. Roizen states that "substituting saturated fat with a healthy fat like olive oil or with nuts . . . decreased heart disease and stroke by 30 percent."

What Roizen fails to note is that olive oil is 11 percent to 14 percent saturated fat – the very artery-clogging fat he advises us to avoid. He also neglects to mention that heart disease is preventable through a whole foods, oil-free plant-based diet. A recent study undertaken by Cleveland Clinic's Dr. Caldwell Esselstyn, published in *The Family Practice Journal*, brings home this point, showing that of those cardiac patients who complied with a whole foods oil-free plant-based diet, only 2.2 percent experienced further cardiac events after 3.7 years compared to the group that did not comply, 62 percent of whose members suffered further cardiac events.

I highly recommend that we take these results to heart (no pun intended) in order to attain optimal health.

Sherry Shrallow

Lincolnshire, Ill.

Posted: Thursday, November 5, 2015 11:00 am

Essy diet can help recovery from heart attack, stroke

Dr. Michael F. Roizen

Special to the CJN

We've talked about how recent headlines indicate you can get a do-over, and that do-over may make you radically younger if you make it to 2024 – and it doesn't take that much to get a do-over if you haven't had structural damage first.

But what if you've already had a heart attack or a stroke. There is good news here for you, but bad news on how many need to take their do-over in two medical reports since July 1, one from The Journal of Family Practice and the second from the Center for Disease Control.

First, Cleveland Clinic's Caldwell Esselstyn, Jr. published a review of 200 consecutive people who visited him for his five-hour course on how to implement his diet to reverse coronary artery disease or at least its symptoms. That this Essy diet ("eat nothing with a face or a mother or added oils," no milk, cheese, eggs, red meat, added olive oil, etc.) or Dr. Dean Ornish's diet can reverse heart disease apparently is not debated in cardiology circles ... just whether people can stay on the diet.

This report and two randomized controlled trials from the Ornish group indicate that that absence of debate about effectiveness may be appropriate ... only one of the 89 percent of people that stayed on the Essy diet suffered a further episode that indicated his arteries were aging, one stroke in the 177 people over 3.7 years.

Most of these 177 had come to Essy because their doc had said there was nothing more they could do for them after multiple stents and coronary artery bypasses and maximal drug therapy did not stop symptoms of inadequate blood flow to their hearts. This would indicate remarkable benefit from this diet, even more so from the Ornish diet that was also successful in preventing progression of cardiac disease.

So to answer the question, can people stay on a diet, Dr. Esselstyn and his team (full disclosure I am on that team) called each person at an average of 3.7 years after they started. The team gathered data on how many of the 200 were still following the diet, and what symptoms they had. Essy was able to reach 198 of the 200, a pretty remarkable number by medical standards for an epidemiologic study. Essy judged after these calls that 177 of the 198 were still strictly following his "eat nothing with a mother, a face or with added oils" diet formula to "Prevent and Reverse Heart Disease" (the name of his book that describes the rationale for the diet and the program in detail).

So 89 percent of these very motivated people could follow the diet and did get relief of symptoms. Could you follow this diet? Well probably less than 20 percent follow any diet they start, so this 89 percent is remarkable, but remember Essy's 200 were motivated. They were having symptoms of progressive aging of arteries in face of prior stents, surgery, and maximal medical therapies. When I started to recommend this to several patients who were in similar situations, I have been surprised that almost all – a notable exception in a ping-pong opponent ¬ have followed the diet strictly at least until their symptoms vanished for six months, and then have liberalized it to once a month fish or salad with olive oil dressing etc. So it is doable.

But even true believers think we need a randomized controlled trial in people who are not so motivated that they visited Essy for a five-hour session on the rationale for the diet, and how to prepare (cook) the diet, to see if even 20 percent of this group can stay with this diet. Till then, should you adopt this or the Ornish diet? The report form the CDC says we as a nation need do something radical in our food choices if we care about our health or even social programs that are being squeezed out by health care.

That report from Essy appeared July 1. The next day the CDC and U.S. Census Bureau teamed up to tell us we need a radical diet change: It pointed out that while aging baby boomers are smoking and drinking less, the vast majority (72 percent of older men and 67 percent of older women) are overweight or obese, which leads to diabetes and arthritis, among other conditions. Further, half of all adults in the US have at least one chronic condition, such as diabetes, heart disease or arthritis. The authors from the CDC add that "chronic diseases are the main causes of poor health, disability, and death, and account for the vast majority (90 percent) of Medicare expenditures. This makes the USA less competitive ... but the paper does point out we are exporting our bad habits – "non-communicable conditions account for nearly two-thirds of deaths worldwide, the emergence of chronic diseases as the predominant challenge to global health is undisputed."

Can a change to a plant based diet like Essy's or Ornish's change these numbers dramatically. Essy and Ornish both believe the answer is yes.

Other reports go on to show that if you enter your Medicare years with five normal (normal waist for height, normal blood pressure, normal blood sugar, normal LDL cholesterol and no cotinine products in your urine (from tobacco) your lifetime Medicare expenditures are 33 percent to 50 percent less, even though you live longer. I think Toby Cosgrove said it best: "The state of our nation is only as good as the state of our nation's health." No doubt we need a diet change if we are to stay strong as a country.

So let's come back to the question, should you try this Essy diet? It makes sense if you have cardiac symptoms or have had need for stents or a coronary artery bypass graft; if you haven't had cardiac or blood vessel dysfunction symptoms yet (remember ED and wrinkles are symptoms or signs or arterial aging) but are at high risk, maybe just modify it to allow salmon, nuts, and olive oil regularly. What's to lose? Most lost weight with the diet. Best, you may keep your arteries young, and learn to spice and enjoy really healthful food, and save enough money from less medical expenditures to enjoy your longer, more energetic life. That way you'll really be a senior, living well.

Dr. Michael F. Roizen is chief wellness officer and chair of the Wellness Institute at Cleveland Clinic.

Here's how I replied:

Posted: Thursday, July 17, 2014 11:00 am

A diet for all

In response to Dr. Michael Roizen's article ("Essy diet can help recovery from heart attack, stroke," July 11), current research does in fact support the role of a whole-foods, plant-based, no-oil diet in the prevention and reversal of heart and vascular disease.

At age 56, I had a heart attack. The day of my emergency bypass surgery, I "coded" three times. I was of normal weight, exercised daily, ate what I thought was a heart-healthy diet and this still happened to me. Had I been eating a whole-foods, plant-based, no-oil diet all along, I know I could have prevented this disease from developing in the first place.

Dr. Roizen is to be commended for advising those with cardiac symptoms and who have had stents or a coronary artery bypass to embrace such a diet. However, I think anyone – even someone who isn't at high risk for heart disease – would be well advised to adopt such a diet. Modification of an animal- and oil-based diet is insufficient in preventing deadly diseases. Eating a plant-based, no-oil diet is.

Please don't wait for heart or vascular disease to appear before changing your lifestyle. Doing so only after a life-threatening event may be too late to act, giving you no second chance to take life-saving preventative measures.

I'm lucky to be alive and will continue to tell my story to help change the way Americans eat so we can all live long, healthy and satisfying lives alongside our loved ones.

Sherry Shrallow

Lincolnshire, Ill.

So you can tell from my remarks to these well respected physicians that there is still a lot of misinformation circulating about what constitutes optimal nutrition. No wonder we are so confused. Isn't it time to pay attention to what the evidence is clearing telling us about the prevention and reversal of heart disease?

16

A New Future for Cardiac Patients

I t is simple.
Nothing comes close to eradicating heart disease as does a plant-based diet.

If you have been diagnosed with cardiovascular disease and are not experiencing a life-threatening cardiac event, your first line of defense should be to establish eating a no-oil WFPD. See how quickly your condition improves, as evidenced by your improved blood work, improved blood flow to your heart and reduction in your blood pressure. Pills and procedures will always be there, and, in some cases, will be necessary, but for most, the results from eating a WFPD will be fast and effective. If your angina pain starts to decrease, know it is from your new way of eating. Let your doctor *see* the results of your arteries opening up through angiograms. Be consistent in your new diet. No cheating with foods that will progress your heart disease. Give it the chance it needs to work for you. I promise you the results will be amazing. Remember, my cholesterol dropped from 175 to 105 in a matter of months!

On my trip with Global Roots to the Dominican Republic in 2015, a woman who was just beginning to eat a WFPD saw her cholesterol drop by 50 points in just one week! If that's not proof of the power of whole foods, I don't know what is.

Thirty minutes spent with cardiologists counseling their patients about the way to eat healthfully will go much further than a 15-minute doctor visit focused on taking vitals and sending us on our way with a renewed prescription. Dr. Esselstyn is a stellar example of what spending time talking to patients can do. In his original study of 17 seriously ill heart patients, he spent time counseling them on their diet every two weeks for five years. He reviewed with them every morsel of food they had eaten, checked their vitals and reported lab results to them to keep them on track. And it worked!

Physicians who use this model of preventive cardiac counseling will see the same results. As a counselor in the mental health field, I understand why this approach works. Therapy is all about the therapeutic relationship I have with my clients. They know I care about their well-being and am devoted to supporting them until they are better. The same goes for medicine. Taking the time to be present with your patients and to listen to, encourage, support and guide them will help them make changes that stick.

We need to continue to establish communities for people who are transitioning to this way of eating so that they have a place to turn to when they need encouragement. That is why I started my cooking classes. We are all in this together and can help each other be well in a fun and relaxing environment.

To be sure, it is difficult to do this on your own. I was forced to because there wasn't a group I could turn to for support. Fortunately, I was the kind of person who was very curious and consequently immersed myself in studies in order to make sound choices about my heart health moving forward. Others, however, may need more structured guidance in terms of adopting this new lifestyle.

Dr. Mike Holly, a physician from Tennessee whom I met at the Global Roots Conference, knows this well. He holds a monthly "Dinner With The Doctor" event where people congregate to enjoy a healthy oil-free plant-based meal and then have the opportunity to ask questions of him and to engage in conversations with others about this lifestyle, many of whom are new to this regime. With his continued support and guidance, he is helping his community make healthful food choices.

There is a man in Detroit, Paul Chatlin, who truly exemplifies the meaning of paying it forward. Paul himself had cardiovascular disease and sought the help of Dr. Caldwell Esselstyn at The Cleveland Clinic. He decided to help others with heart disease by creating an organization in Detroit called Plant Based Nutrition Support Group. His group provides education and support for all of those in his area who are living the plant-based lifestyle. He and Dr. Joel Kahn, a local cardiologist, have partnered to bring in world-class speakers and have arranged outings to restaurants where the food is totally plant-based and oil-free. Paul has made a significant difference in his community, turning his own experience with heart disease from lemons to lemonade. Paul and I chatted on the phone briefly many years ago when he was just getting started with his group. His passion as he spoke about wanting to eradicate this disease came through loud and clear.. We surely need more Paul Chatlins in this world.

In recent years, the plant-based movement has been gaining momentum and is nothing short of a revolution today. Think back to the civil rights movement, the fight against smoking and other noble causes whose primary existence was to right a wrong. It took years and years for these movements to take hold, but take hold they did. Thank goodness, we are now seeing it in the area of plant-based nutrition, something that can help everyone lead a healthy and happy life.

My plea is for doctors to honor their commitment to do no harm and as Hippocrates, the Father of Medicine, said, "Let food be thy medicine and medicine be thy food."

And finally, I wish good health and happy, peaceful lives to all. Let's get there together.

17

How to Transition to a WFPD - A New Beginning

Moving away from the standard American diet and towards a no-oil WFPD can be a bit daunting at first. Change is hard. No other way around it. Change, however, is possible. Here are some helpful tips I found along the way when transitioning to this new way of living.

When I decided to go plant-based, I started in my kitchen. I took everything out of my refrigerator, freezer and pantry and put in one pile the foods I could keep and in another those I had to dispose of. Once I packed all the unwanted foods and gave them away, I saw how little was left in my kitchen.

The next step was to go to the grocery store and start buying as much fresh produce as I could along with other staples. (I am including a "How to Stock My Plant-based Kitchen" guide in chapter 18 to guide your grocery shopping for your new pantry items.)

Going to the grocery store to find foods that were safe for me to eat was challenging, to say the least. Looking at labels is the key. As I wrote earlier, making sure to check the oil, sodium, and sugar content on labels is vital. You want to avoid any product that contains oil, which, unfortunately, predominates the shelves. In my guide, I have listed some "safe" products currently on the market for you to consider.

My next step was to start trying out recipes. I began with Ann Esselstyn's recipes in the book *Prevent and Reverse Heart Disease*.[39] They were delicious, and I still have certain favorites, such as Lentil Joes, which you can find in my freezer on a regular basis. Over the years many more cookbooks have come out that I use regularly. For those like me who love to cook, I have a blast trying new things. However, when you are just starting out, don't feel as if you must become a gourmet chef to eat this way. You really don't. Keeping things simple will keep you on track. For example, for dinner, after a hard day's work, I might come home and take out some corn tortillas that I have in my freezer (make sure they contain no oil). I then line a large baking sheet with parchment paper. I place the tortillas on the sheet and open up a can of no-sodium black beans and corn. I rinse them and then place the beans and corn on top of the tortillas. I might top it with salsa or with some pico de gallo and then bake them at 350 degrees for 15-20 minutes and then, voilà, dinner is served! While they're baking, I would toss a salad and make my own dressing by mixing balsamic vinegar with equal parts of one of my favorite mustards (I love dijon) and a teaspoonful of maple syrup and there's my salad dressing. This is a nutritious and delicious meal done in less than 30 minutes.

Having about six regular dinners you can make and feel comfortable with is a good start. As you continue to eat this way you will find yourself adding more ideas to your go to meals. I'll share with you in a Chapter 19 my very favorite recipes that you can start making in your own kitchen today.

Another very easy go to dinner is a stir fry. All you need to do is to cook some rice when you come home from work and, while it's cooking, cut up veggies you love for your stir fry. I use mushrooms, broccoli, carrots, bok choy, green onions, red peppers, or whatever else I have in the refrigerator that I'm in the mood for. As I learned from Chef Del Sroufe, stir fry your vegetables in small amounts of water or fat-free vegetable broth so that the vegetables stay crisp and don't stick to the fry pan. This takes only about 5-10 minutes. Start with onions first and then add the remaining vegetables. Add stir fry sauce, mix all together and dinner is served. You can also add some non-GMO tofu as well if you'd like; all you have to do is cut the tofu into small squares and add them to your skillet at the end of stir frying so that they get steamed through.

Soups, chilis and casseroles are another great way to have food ready when you need it. I created an amazing vegetable, bean and miso soup, that I keep frozen and ready to eat at a moment's notice. Ann Esselstyn's split pea soup is another favorite of mine. Chili and casseroles are both easy to put together and so satisfying to eat.

I usually whip up a few entrees on the weekend that I know I can freeze and then go to when it's dinnertime. That way I am never tempted to eat unhealthy foods (plus I don't keep the wrong things in my house anymore).

For breakfast, I eat oatmeal every day, made with my homemade almond milk. To my oatmeal bowl I add a tablespoon of flaxseed, ¼ teaspoon turmeric and a cup of blueberries. It is so good! I feel deprived if I can't have it. Lunch is simple too. I put hummus (that I make myself) on a whole wheat wrap and add fresh veggies like spinach, kale, tomatoes, cucumbers and peppers and have a great treat. I also make great salads I can carry to work. One of my favorites is a kale salad recipe I use that I could eat for breakfast, lunch or dinner. Soups that you make and freeze into individual containers are another go to for lunch.

Whole grain, rice, quinoa or spelt pastas with a no-oil store marinara sauce or my own homemade cauliflower or potato/carrot sauce likewise make for quick meals. So, you're getting the idea. Start with a few tasty recipes in your repertoire and go from there.

You may be wondering about desserts. I love desserts but have to limit them to special occasions. Sugar is not our best friend. Sweets (like oils) are very addicting and not doing your body any good if eaten on a regular basis. If you must have something sweet, consider freezing grapes and enjoying them or making banana "ice cream."

Enjoy your meals and eat as much as you like, and don't be afraid of the rice and potatoes. Dr. John McDougall, who wrote *The Starch Solution*, has long been singing the praises of these foods, which are eaten by most people around the world. They are filling and satisfying. Remember, this is not a diet but a lifestyle, and one filled with abundance. You will never be hungry and find it easier to indulge in sweets only occasionally when filling up on starches, legumes, fruits and vegetables.

On the subject of diets, while eating this way you will most likely see your weight go down. Here's why. Calories from plants are burned off more quickly and not stored in the body as fat as are animal foods. Dr. T. Colin Campbell discusses this phenomenon in *The China Study*:

> Average calorie intake, per kilogram of body weight, was 30% higher among the least active Chinese than among average Americans. Yet, their body weight was 20% lower.

He goes on to say, "Provided that we aren't restricting our calorie intake, those of us who consume a high-fat, high protein diet simply retain more calories than we need. We store these calories as body fat, perhaps weave it into our muscle fibers (we call it "marbling" in beef animals) and perhaps store it in the more obvious places, like our butt, our midsection or around our face and upper thighs."

He concludes with: "This is what our China Study data show. Chinese consume more calories both because they are more physically active and because their consumption of low-fat, low-protein diets shifts conversion of these calories away from body fat to body heat."[40]

The only way one can gain weight eating plant-based is if you partake in what I like to call processed vegan junk foods, like potato chips, vegan pastries, and foods loaded with oil. This is not what a WFPD looks like.

As I mentioned earlier, it is imperative if you have Type 2 diabetes to consult with your doctor when transitioning to the WFPD because your blood sugar levels will improve rapidly and will necessitate a medication reevaluation and readjustment (less medication over time will be needed). Some may come off their diabetes medications altogether.

The easiest way to move towards eating this way is to join a group and have fun with your food. Find a group that cooks together or a social group that dines out together and get involved. A good place to start your search wherever you live is through Meetup.com. If a group doesn't exist in your area, start one as I did. The cost is minimal and you'll be helping others on their journey. You will meet the nicest people and have something in common right off the bat. You also won't feel isolated or alone. Our numbers are growing but we are still a minority group in this country.

I would also advise to look for educational opportunities to expand your knowledge on plant-based nutrition. As I said earlier, I read books, watched documentaries, and eventually enrolled in the certificate program at the T. Colin Campbell Center for Nutrition Studies through e-Cornell University. There are so many other excellent training programs available as well. One is through the Wellness Forum in Columbus, Ohio, run by Dr. Pamela Popper. Dr. John McDougall also offers a training program through his Wellness Center in

Santa Rosa, California, as does the Physicians Committee for Responsible Medicine.

You can also take chef training courses to advance your skills in the kitchen. One such program is offered by the Forks over Knives organization, available online.

There are also opportunities to learn from the world's leading experts on plant-based nutrition while on vacation: Dr. John McDougall's trips in Hawaii and Costa Rica, Holistic Holidays at Sea Caribbean cruises, and LeAnne Campbell's Global Roots conferences in the Dominican Republic, just to name a couple.

Online programs to facilitate transitioning to a WFPD, through their kick-start challenges are also available. Organizations that offer them include The Physician's Committee for Responsible Medicine, Rip Esselstyn's Engine 2, and PlantPure Nation.

You can also subscribe to online newsletters from Dr. Pamela Popper, Dr. John McDougall, Dr. Neal Barnard, and Dr. Michael Greger, each providing the most up-to-date scientific information about diet and disease prevention. These are all free resources available to you.

Remember earlier I addressed the often asked question "Where do you get your protein?" Here's what you can say. Just tell them that all the whole foods you eat contain protein and that you get just the right amount of protein when you eat this way. Sort of laugh with them and say, "Can you believe fruits and vegetables, legumes and whole grains all contain protein and nobody told us? And the best part is they don't contain any cholesterol so I can't build up plaque in my arteries! Isn't that amazing?"

When I started out on my journey I had some business cards printed that read *Staying Alive*. Yes, staying alive was my goal when I first recovered from my heart attack and bypass surgery but it means so much more than that to me now. Staying alive for me means living life to its fullest and being of service to others by giving back what I have learned. If I can do that and have reached you by writing about my own experience with heart disease, then I'm a happy camper.

As my dear yoga teacher and friend says at the end of each of our yoga practices, "May you be happy and know the roots of your happiness. May you be safe from inner and outer harm. May you be free from pain and suffering and may your life unfold with ease." I send this out to you and leave you with one word that is said at the end of all yoga practices.

Namaste. May the light within me bow to and honor the light within you.

18

How to Stock Your Plant-based Kitchen

COOKING EQUIPMENT

Set of non-stick pots and pans
Measuring cups and measuring spoons
Mixing spoons
Whisk
Spatula
Soup ladle
Grater
Nut bag (to make homemade plant milks)
Rolling pin
Strainers
Mixing bowls of various sizes
Lemon juicer
Set of good knives for slicing and dicing
Cutting boards
Can opener
Casserole pans (8x8 and 9x11)

Loaf pan

Parchment paper (you'll use this on your baking sheets and baking dishes)

Vitamix blender (or any other high-powered blender)

Food processer

Crock pot slow cooker

Instant Pot or any good Pressure Cooker

Air Fryer by Philips (I don't have one yet but I hear great things about it from my friends)

Rice cooker

Storage containers to freeze foods

FOODS:

Start with what you need and add on slowly.

Fruits – all kinds (avoid or limit coconuts if you have heart disease). Always keep medjool dates on hand to use in homemade almond milk.

Vegetables – include leafy green vegetables, root vegetables, red, purple, orange and yellow vegetables, avoiding or limiting avocados if you have heart disease because of their high fat content. Always have lots of onions and garlic on hand. I cook with them regularly.

Legumes – alfalfa, asparagus bean, asparagus pea bean, baby lima bean, black bean, black-eyed peas, black turtle bean, Boston bean, Boston navy bean, broad bean, cannellini bean, chickpeas, chili bean, cranberry bean, dwarf bean, Egyptian bean, Egyptian white broad bean, English bean, fava bean, fava coceira, field pea, French green bean, Frijol Bola Roja, frijole negro, great northern bean, green bean, green and yellow peas, kidney bean, lentils (red, brown and green), lespedeza, licorice, lima bean, Madagascar bean, Mexican black bean, Mexican red bean, molasses face bean, mung bean, mung pea, navy bean, pea bean, peanut, Peruvian bean, pinto bean, red bean, red clover, red eye bean, red kidney bean, rice bean, runner bean, scarlet runner bean, small red bean, snow pea, southern pea, sugar snap pea, soybean, wax bean, white kidney bean, white pea bean

Whole grains – whole wheat pasta, breads (Ezekiel 4:9 sprouted grain breads, buns and tortillas), Engine 2 Plant-Strong Sprouted Ancient Grain tortillas, or their gluten-free variety made with rice flour, Whole Foods brand fat free tortillas. Read labels on other brands to check for oil. Most breads have oil listed as one of their ingredients.

Vegetable Broth – Pacific brand low sodium, oil-free.

Cereals – Organic oat meals (Bob's Red Mill is my favorite), Grape Nuts cereal, Post shredded wheat and bran, Engine 2 Plant-Strong cereals at Whole Foods, Whole Foods bite-size wheat cereal.

Crackers – Whole Foods 365 Woven Wheats baked crackers, Engine 2 crackers, Mary's Gone Crackers organic, gluten free whole grain crackers, unsalted whole wheat matzo crackers

Hummus/Spreads/Dips – Whole Foods low-fat hummus, Whole Foods mango salsa and pineapple salsa, Engine 2 Plant-Strong Hummus (several varieties to choose from)

Sorbet – Dole sorbet in fruit flavors, Dreyer's whole-fruit bars, Eddy's whole fruit products

Pasta Sauce – Engine 2 brand, Whole Foods low fat pasta sauce, Muir Glen Organic Portobello Mushroom pasta sauce

Stir Fry Sauce – Annie Chun's Gourmet Shitake Soy Ginger Sauce (no oil and low sodium, at Whole Foods)

Diced Tomatoes – no salt

Tomato Sauce and Tomato Paste – no salt

Mustards – dijon, horseradish mustard, yellow, stone-ground and spicy brown

Jelly (low sugar varieties)

Horseradish

Vinegars – apple cider, white, balsamic, rice and all other flavors for salad dressings. I buy mine from *The Olive Tap*. Can have them shipped.

Vegan Worcestershire sauce

Liquid Smoke

Spike seasoning (a salt substitute)

Miso Paste – made from soy and comes in white and red; look for low sodium variety

Chickpea Miso – gluten-free version of miso

Butler Soy Curls – order on Amazon

Non-GMO Tofu – comes in extra firm, firm and silken

Tempeh – fermented soy product

Brag Liquid Aminos

Low Sodium Tamari and Soy Sauce

Ener G Egg Replacer

Flours – whole wheat, whole wheat pastry flour, barley, buckwheat, chickpea, brown rice, and oat flours

Grains – barley, bulgur, corn, farro, kamut, millet, oats, popcorn, quinoa, rice, rye, sorghum, spelt, teff, wild rice. When buying rice look for ones grown in California- they contain less arsenic.

Vital Wheat Gluten

Nuts – pine, walnuts, almonds, pecans (limit if you have heart disease)

Seeds – chia, hemp, pomegranate, flax (buy ground or grind yourself), poppy, pumpkin, apricot, sesame, sunflower, cumin, and grape seeds

Peanut Butter and Almond Butter – use limited amounts of fresh ground that you can get at Whole Foods (limit if you have heart disease)

Ketchup – look for brands without corn syrup

BBQ Sauce – I buy Russ & Frank brand at Whole Foods; it has very low sodium, is oil-free and is very tasty

Relish –I buy McClure's brand at Whole Foods because it has no preservatives

Nutritional Yeast

Corn Meal

Organic Cane Sugar

Sucanat

Brown Sugar

Powdered Sugar

Light Agave Nectar

Maple Syrup

Cornstarch

Arrowroot Powder

Tapioca

Baking Soda

Baking Powder

Molasses

Cocoa powder

Carob powder

Enjoy Life Dairy-Free Chocolate Chips

Pure vanilla extract, almond extract, peppermint extract

Pure vanilla bean paste

Espresso powder

PB 2 powdered peanut butter

Applesauce

Spring Roll Skins

Canned Artichokes

Fresh herbs – parsley, cilantro, basil, thyme and rosemary

Spices – allspice, basil, bay leaves, cayenne pepper, cardamom, chipotle chili, chili powder, cinnamon, cloves, coriander, cumin seeds, curry, fennel, garlic powder, ginger powder, ground mace, marjoram, mustard seed, nutmeg, onion powder, oregano, paprika, pumpkin pie seasoning, smoked paprika, parsley, black pepper, vegan poultry seasoning, rosemary, sage, salt, thyme, turmeric, white pepper, Spike seasoning

Panko Bread Crumbs – Ian's brand is oil-free; comes in whole wheat, original and gluten-free

Plant Milks- soy (I use Westsoy Organic Unsweetened Plain, just soybeans and water, no preservatives), almond, hemp, oat and rice

Non-caffeinated teas (Hibiscus is wonderful for lowering blood pressure naturally)

19

My Favorite Plant-Based Recipes

BREAKFAST

FRENCH TOAST

created by Mary McDougall in
The Starch Solution and adapted by Sherry Shrallow

Ingredients:

2 cups homemade almond milk

1/8 teaspoon ground cinnamon

Dash of ground turmeric

12 slices whole wheat bread

Directions:

1. Add all ingredients to a large bowl and mix thoroughly. Dip slices of bread in it, one at a time, coating well.

2. Heat nonstick skillet over medium heat. Cook each piece until nicely browned on each side and serve warm with toppings of your choice.

ALMOND MILK

created by Sherry Shrallow

Directions:

Soak 1 cup of raw almonds in cold water for 4-6 hours. Drain almonds and rinse thoroughly. Place in Vitamix blender along with 4 ½ cups of cold water, a splash of vanilla and 4 medjool dates, pitted.

Blend on high speed for about 2 minutes. Pour mixture into a large bowl through a nut bag. Squeeze liquid through into the bowl and discard the almond paste left in the nut bag. Pour your almond milk into a pitcher and store in refrigerator for 2-3 days.

GREEN PEPPER TOFU SCRAMBLE

created by Kim Campbell in
The PlantPure Nation Cookbook

Prep: 15 minutes Cook: 10 minutes Servings: 4

Ingredients:

1 onion, diced

1 green bell pepper, seeded and diced medium

½ jalapeno pepper, seeded and minced

¼ cup low-sodium vegetable stock, for sautéing

¼ teaspoon ground turmeric

2 tablespoons nutritional yeast flakes

1 tablespoon garlic powder

¼ teaspoon sea salt

¼ teaspoon black pepper

2 tablespoons Bragg Liquid Aminos

One 14-ounce block extra firm tofu, drained and crumbled

3 tablespoons chopped parsley (optional)

Directions:

1. In a skillet over medium-high heat, sauté the onion, bell pepper, and jalapeño pepper in

the vegetable stock. Cook for 5 minutes, or until the vegetables become tender.

2. Stir in the spices and soy sauce. Continue cooking for 1-2 minutes.

3. Add the crumbled tofu and turn the heat to low. Cook for an additional 1-2 minutes.

4. Remove from the heat and stir in the fresh parsley, if using. Serve immediately.

STEEL CUT OATMEAL WITH FLAXSEEDS AND FIXINGS

created by Sherry Shrallow

I make this recipe in my Instant Pot pressure cooker with enough to last for 4 days.

Ingredients:

1 cup steel cut oats

3 cups Sherry's homemade almond milk

1 tablespoon flaxseeds

¼ teaspoon turmeric

1 cup blueberries (I use frozen organic from Costco and microwave for 1-2 minutes)

Any greens, or other fruits you like

Directions:

Add your milk and oats into your Instant Pot pressure cooker. Do not stir the oats. Set manual cooking and adjust timer to 3 minutes on high pressure. Seal lid and wait until done. Let steam release naturally for about 25 minutes. Put one portion of cooked oatmeal in bowl along with blueberries, flaxseed, greens and turmeric.

CHICKPEA FLOUR OMELETS WITH ASPARAGUS

created by Susan Voisin at fatfreevegan.com

Ingredients:

8 ounces of asparagus, ends trimmed and stalks cut into 1-inch pieces

½ cup superfine chickpea four

2 tablespoons nutritional yeast

1 tablespoon ground flax or chia seeds

1 teaspoon dried basil

½ teaspoon baking powder

¼ teaspoon turmeric

¼ teaspoon salt

1/8 teaspoon black salt (kala namak) – optional, but gives an "eggy" flavor

Generous grinding of black pepper to taste

¾ cup water

1 tablespoon fresh chives, snipped (or 1 tablespoon minced onion)

½ green or red bell pepper, chopped

1 small tomato, chopped, or a handful of halved grape tomatoes, optional

Instructions:

1. Cook the asparagus until it is tender by steaming or roasting in 425 degree oven for about 10 minutes. Sprinkle with salt to taste, if you like, and set aside.

2. Mix the chickpea flour with all dry ingredients (nutritional yeast through black pepper) in a medium mixing bowl. Add the water, chives, and bell pepper. Allow to stand and thicken while the asparagus cooks about 10 minutes.

3. Check the batter and add water by the tablespoon if it is not a pourable consistency. It should be like thick pancake batter.

4. Preheat a large non-stick skillet or cast iron skillet over high heat. Once it's hot, reduce the heat to medium and pour half of the

batter (about 2/3 cup) into the center of the skillet. Smooth it with the back of a spoon until it's a circle about 6 inches in diameter. If you're using tomatoes, sprinkle half of them on top. Cover tightly and cook for 4 minutes or until the top begins to look bread-like rather than liquidy.

5. Add half the asparagus to one side of the omelet and fold the other half over it. Cover and cook for another 3-4 minutes. Repeat with remaining ingredients for one more omelet. Serve warm.

THE BEST BANANA BREAD

created by Ann Crile Esselstyn in
Prevent and Reverse Heart Disease

Ingredients:

1 ¼ cup whole-wheat flour

1 cup barley or spelt flour

1 teaspoon baking powder

1 teaspoon baking soda

1 teaspoon ground cinnamon

3 small ripe bananas, or 2 large

1 jar baby food prunes, or ½ cup applesauce

1/3 cup (or less) maple syrup, honey or sugar

Egg replacer for 1 egg (1 tablespoon ground flaxseed meal mixed with 3 tablespoons water) OR

½ teaspoon Ener-G egg replacer mixed with 2 tablespoons water

½ cup raisins

2 teaspoons vanilla extract

¾ cup any nonfat plant milk (I use my homemade almond milk, but soy, oat or multigrain is fine as well)

1 tablespoon lemon juice

Directions:

1. Preheat oven to 350 degrees.

2. Mix first 5 ingredients into a large bowl.

3. Mash bananas in a medium bowl. Mix in remaining ingredients with bananas.

4. Add liquids to flour and mix gently. Pour into a 9 x 5-inch loaf pan and bake for 70 minutes, until a toothpick comes out clean.

SALADS AND DRESSINGS

TRANSCENDENT TABBOULEH

created by Wendy Solganik at Healthy Girls Kitchen

Ingredients:

¾ cup bulgur

1 cup boiling water

3 cups finely chopped fresh parsley

Heaping ¼ cup fresh mint, finely chopped

Heaping ¼ cup finely chopped scallions

2 plum (Italian) tomatoes, finely diced

1 cup cucumber, finely diced

2-3 cloves garlic, finely minced

2 tablespoons fresh lemon juice

½ teaspoon cumin

½ teaspoon salt

¼ teaspoon black pepper

Directions:

1. Place bulgur in a medium bowl and cover with the boiling water.

2. Seal bowl and let sit until the water is absorbed and the bulgur is tender, about 15 minutes.

3. Place all other ingredients into a large bowl and add the cooked bulgur. Toss to combine.

SHERRY'S FAT-FREE POTATO SALAD

created by Sherry Shrallow

Ingredients:

6 red potatoes, diced into the size you'd like for your salad

½ onion, minced

¼ cup apple cider vinegar

1 tablespoon dijon mustard

1 teaspoon maple syrup

2 tablespoons fresh dill

Directions:

1. Boil potatoes for about 20 minutes, until tender (not too soft)

2. Drain potatoes and place in large mixing bowl.

3. Add remaining ingredients and mix gently until combined. Can eat warm or place in refrigerator until chilled.

4. Note. Taste sauce before pouring over potatoes to get it just right for you. Adjust seasonings accordingly.

TOFU EGGLESS "EGG-LIKE" SALAD

from Helyn's plant-based kitchen (http:helynskitchen.com)

Ingredients:

1 ½ cups raw cashews, soaked for about 5 hours (or overnight is fine)

About ½ cup water

2 tablespoons yellow mustard

½ teaspoon onion powder

½ teaspoon curry powder

½ teaspoon turmeric powder

½ teaspoon black salt (kala namak), gives salad a distinctive eggy flavor

1 package extra- firm silken tofu

Directions:

1. Rinse the cashews and place in a high-powered blender. Add water a little at a time, blending until you reach a smooth, pasty consistency.

2. Add the remaining ingredients, except the tofu, and blend again until combined.

3. Transfer to a bowl and crumble in the tofu.

4. Fold in gently to combine.

Add chopped onions, celery or anything else you like.

CHICKPEA SALAD WITH ORANGE MISO DRESSING

created by Leslie Haas

Salad Ingredients:

12 cherry tomatoes, halved

4 green onions, sliced

½ cup dry quinoa (cook according to package directions)

1 ½ cups chickpeas, cooked or canned and rinsed

3 tablespoons fresh cilantro

Dressing Ingredients:

¼ cup fresh orange juice (juice of 2 oranges)

¼ cup seasoned rice vinegar

2 teaspoons white or yellow miso

1 tablespoon maple syrup or agave nectar

1 clove garlic, grated or minced

1 teaspoon ginger, grated or minced

2 teaspoons black (or white) sesame seeds

Directions:

1. Combine the tomatoes, onions, quinoa, chickpeas, and fresh cilantro in a large bowl.

2. Mix the dressing ingredients together in a small bowl.

3. Pour the dressing into the larger bowl and toss all of the salad ingredients together.

(Leslie's tip: a high power blender for the dressing eliminates the need to mince the ginger and garlic and distributes the flavors nicely throughout the salad! I blend with the vinegar, etc., then gently stir in the orange juice and fold in the sesame seeds as the dressing is mixed in.)

KALE SALAD WITH MAPLE-MUSTARD DRESSING

created by Julieanna Hever in
Forks Over Knives - The Cookbook and
adapted by Sherry Shrallow

Serves 4 to 6

Ingredients for the Dressing:

One 15-ounce can cannellini beans, drained and rinsed

2 tablespoons stone-ground or dijon mustard

2 tablespoons nutritional yeast

1 tablespoon low-sodium soy sauce or Bragg Liquid Aminos

1 tablespoon 100% pure maple syrup

Zest and juice of 1 lemon

¼ cup water

Ingredients for the Salad:

6 cups kale, massaged for 5 minutes and then shredded

1 cup shredded red cabbage

1 cup shredded carrots

1 cup finely chopped broccoli florets

One 15-ounce can chickpeas, drained and rinsed

1/3 cup low sugar Craisins

1. To make the dressing: In blender, add all dressing ingredients and blend until smooth. Add water if too thick.

2. To make the salad: Add all ingredients into a large bowl and toss with dressing.

JANE'S FAVORITE 3, 2, 1 DRESSING

created by Jane Esselstyn in
The Prevent and Reverse Heart Disease Cookbook

Ingredients:

3 tablespoons balsamic vinegar

2 tablespoons mustard of your choice

1 tablespoon pure maple syrup

Juice of 1 lemon

Pinch of freshly ground white pepper (optional)

Directions:

Combine all ingredients in a small bowl with a whisk until smooth.

NUTMEG NOTEBOOK CREAMY BALSAMIC DRESSING

created by Tami Kramer from tami@nutmegnotebooks.com

Ingredients:

1 box or can of cannellini beans no salt added, rinsed and drained

½ cup balsamic vinegar

4 medjool dates

4 teaspoons dijon mustard

1 cup unsweetened plant milk

2 cloves fresh garlic

Directions:

Mix all in Vitamix blender until smooth and creamy. It thickens when refrigerated.

DALE'S DRESSING

created by my dear husband Dale Shrallow

Ingredients:

1 tablespoon dijon mustard

¾ teaspoon white horseradish

1 ½ teaspoons balsamic vinegar

Directions:

Whisk together and done!

SOUPS

BUTTERNUT SQUASH SOUP

created by Sherry Shrallow

Ingredients:

2-3 pounds butternut squash, peeled and cut into 1 inch chunks

3 large carrots, chopped

1 medium onion, chopped

2 quarts vegetable broth (I use low sodium Pacific brand vegetable broth or make my own)

1 bunch of dill or parsley (I prefer the dill)

Pinch of nutmeg

Salt and freshly ground pepper to taste

Tony Chachere's Original Creole seasoning to taste (gives the soup a "kick")

Directions:

1. Put all ingredients in a pot and bring to a boil.
2. Simmer for 1 hour.

3. Puree soup with hand-held immersion blender or put in high powered blender (I use a Vitamix) until smooth and creamy.

VEGETABLE BEAN AND MISO SOUP

created by Sherry Shrallow

Ingredients:

2 boxes of low sodium, fat free vegetable broth (Pacific Brand)

1 onion, chopped and diced

2-3 carrots, cut into small pieces

2-3 stalks celery, chopped into small pieces

1 parsnip, peeled, and cut into small pieces

1 large potato, peeled and cut into cubes

½ cup farro

1 can diced tomatoes

1 tablespoon dried fennel

1 can low sodium corn, drained

1 can kidney beans, rinsed and drained

1 can cannellini beans, rinsed and drained

½ cup frozen peas

Fresh parsley

White miso, to taste

Directions:

1. Place all ingredients in a large soup pot except for the white miso and bring to a boil.

2. Lower heat and cook at least one hour, simmering on a low boil.

3. When done, take off heat.

4. Mix 1-2 tablespoons miso with hot water until pasty.

5. Add to soup pot and stir in until blended.

6. Taste to see if more is needed.

SWEET POTATO, SWISS CHARD AND RED LENTIL SOUP

created by Del Sroufe in The China Study Family Cookbook

Red lentils are one of the quickest cooking legumes and one of the most flavorful.

Serves 12

Ingredients:

4-6 cups of low sodium vegetable broth (start with 4 cups and add more as needed)

1 ½ large yellow onions, diced

3 stalks celery, diced

3 large carrots, peeled and diced

6 cloves garlic, minced

1 ½ tablespoons ground cumin

3/8 teaspoon ground allspice

3 cups red lentils

1 ½ large sweet potatoes, peeled and diced

1 ½ large bunch swiss chard, chopped

Sea salt and black pepper to taste

Juice of 1 ½ lemons

Directions:

1. Sauté the onion, celery and carrots in a large saucepan over medium heat until the onions are translucent and start to brown.

2. Add water 1 to 2 tablespoons at a time to keep the vegetables from sticking.

3. Add the garlic, cumin, and allspice, and cook another minute.

4. Add the vegetable broth, lentils, and sweet potato. Bring the pot to a boil over high heat, reduce the heat to medium and simmer the soup for 20 minutes until the sweet potatoes and lentils are tender.

5. Add the swiss chard, season with salt and pepper and cook another 10 minutes until the chard is cooked.

6. Add the lemon juice, mix well and serve.

CREAM OF POTATO MUSHROOM AND DILL SOUP

created by Chef Del Sroufe

Serves 6-8

Ingredients:

2 leeks, chopped

2 large carrots, sliced

6 cups Pacific brand low-sodium vegetable broth

2 teaspoons dried dill weed

2 teaspoons sea salt (I use half of this and then add to your bowl if needed)

2 pounds of potatoes, peeled and diced

1 pound fresh mushrooms, sliced

1 cup unsweetened plant milk

3 tablespoons arrow root powder

Fresh dill weed for garnish (optional)

Directions:

1. Sauté the leeks, carrots, and mushrooms in a large saucepan over medium heat for 8 minutes. Add the vegetable broth, dill, sea salt, and potatoes. Cover, and cook 20

minutes or until the potatoes are tender but firm.

2. In a small bowl, mix the plant milk and arrow root powder until smooth. Stir into the soup to thicken.

3. Garnish each bowl with fresh dill if you'd like.

SPLIT PEA SOUP

created by Ann Crile Esselstyn in Prevent and Reverse Heart Disease

Ingredients:

3 cups dry split peas

8 cups water (can add more water if you think soup is too thick)

1 bay leaf

1 teaspoon dry mustard

1 large onion, chopped (1 cup)

4-5 medium garlic cloves, crushed

3 ribs celery, freshly chopped (3/4 cup)

3 medium carrots, sliced or diced

5 small potatoes, sliced, then cut like french fries

Freshly ground black pepper

3-4 tablespoons red wine vinegar or balsamic vinegar

1 large ripe tomato, diced (one cup)

Lots of chopped cilantro or parsley

Directions:

1. Place split peas, water, bay leaf, and mustard in a heavy soup pot. Bring to a boil, lower heat, and simmer, partially covered, for about 20 minutes,

2. Add onion, garlic, celery, carrots, and potatoes. Cover and simmer for about 40 minutes, stirring occasionally. Add water if soup is too thick. When done, add freshly ground black pepper, vinegar, and top with diced tomatoes and cilantro or parsley.

CREAMY CELERIAC SOUP

created by Susan Voisin at fatfreevegan.com

Ingredients:

1 large, or 2 medium celery roots (4-5 cups chopped)

1 medium onion, chopped

4 cloves garlic, peeled

3 cups Pacific brand low sodium vegetable broth, divided

1/8 teaspoon white pepper (or to taste)

½ teaspoon thyme

½ teaspoon salt (or to taste)

¼ cup non-dairy milk

½ teaspoon lemon juice

Directions:

1. Peel the celery root and cut into equal-sized cubes (about ¾ inch).

2. In large saucepan, sauté the onion and whole garlic until the onion begins to brown. Add the celery root and 2 cups of the vegetable broth.

3. Pour cooked celeriac and remaining broth into a Vitamix blender and puree, starting at low speed and increasing to high, in batches until completely smooth. Take care when blending because hot liquids can erupt from the blender and cause serious burns. Never fill your blender more than half full. Also, remove the center cup on the two-part lid and cover the opening with a kitchen towel to allow hot air to escape and prevent pressure from building up.

4. Pour back into the pot and add white pepper, thyme, and salt.

5. Simmer for 15-20 minutes, adding additional broth if the soup gets too thick.

6. Add non-dairy milk and lemon juice, stir well, and simmer for 5 more minutes.

7. Add more salt and pepper to taste and serve hot.

APPETIZERS

SPICY CAULIFLOWER HOT WINGS

Adapted by Sherry Shrallow from numerous recipes

Ingredients:

1 head cauliflower

1 cup whole wheat flour

½ cup corn meal

1 cup water or unsweetened almond milk

1 teaspoon onion powder

1 teaspoon garlic powder

¼ cup nutritional yeast

1 cup breadcrumbs or panko bread crumbs

¾ teaspoon Spike seasoning (salt substitute)

½ cup barbecue sauce

Tabasco sauce to taste (few drops)

Directions:

1. Whisk flour and water or milk in large bowl. Cut cauliflower into small florets. Add to flour mixture and coat evenly.

2. Dip into second large mixing bowl that contains the bread crumbs, corn meal, onion powder, garlic powder, nutritional yeast and salt substitute.

3. Place each floret on baking sheet lined with parchment paper and bake at 450 degrees for 15-20 minutes, or until crispy and browned.

4. Remove florets from baking sheet and add to a large bowl containing the barbecue sauce and tabasco sauce. Coat evenly and return to baking sheet lined with parchment paper. Bake an additional 20 minutes.

OUR HUMMUS

created by Ann Crile Esselstyn and Jane Esselstyn in
The Prevent and Reverse Heart Disease Cookbook

Ingredients:

One 15-ounce can salt-free chickpeas, drained and rinsed

2 large cloves garlic

2 tablespoons fresh lemon juice

1 ½ tablespoons spicy brown mustard, or to taste

Freshly ground black pepper, to taste

¼ teaspoon salt (optional)

Directions:

In a food processor, combine the all ingredients and 2 tablespoons water, and process until uniformly smooth.

SWEET AND SAVORY MINI LATKES

contributed by Kenden Alfond at Jewish Food Hero

Ingredients:

1 large sweet potato (or yam), peeled and coarsely grated

1 parsnip, peeled and coarsely grated

¼ cup all-purpose flour or gluten free all-purpose flour

¼ teaspoon baking soda

½ teaspoon sea salt

¼ teaspoon black pepper

3 tablespoons cooked sweet potato

1 tablespoon low fat non-dairy milk

Large mixing bowl

Baking sheet lined with parchment paper

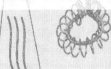

For Tofu Sour "Cream"

1 cup silken tofu

1-2 teaspoons lemon juice

¼ teaspoon sea salt

2 tablespoons minced fresh chives

Blend ingredients for this Tofu Sour "Cream" in a food processor or blender.

Directions:

1. Preheat oven to 350 degrees.

2. In a large mixing bowl, place grated raw sweet potato and parsnip.

3. Add flour, baking soda, sea salt, black pepper and 3 tablespoons of the mashed sweet potato. Stir to combine. Add the non-dairy milk.

4. On parchment lined baking sheet, scoop up a rounded tablespoon of the latke mixture and form it into a ball with your hands. Flatten slightly to create a little patty. Repeat with remaining mixture. Makes 16.

5. Bake for 25 minutes, or until golden on one side. Flip the latkes gently.

6. Bake for another 15 minutes or until golden brown.

7. Serve with tofu sour "cream" and applesauce.

MUSHROOM CABBAGE POTSTICKERS

contributed by Whitney Ross and
Rebecca Clayman at whitneyross@mac.com

Makes 55 to 60 pot stickers

Pot sticker Ingredients:

4 ounces mushrooms, stems removed and caps diced small

1 pound Napa cabbage

1 teaspoon sea salt

6-7 ounces firm tofu

1 tablespoon minced ginger

1 clove garlic, minced

1 ½ tablespoons rice vinegar

1 tablespoon tamari

½ teaspoon black pepper

55 to 60 circular or square-shaped (4.5 inches) dumpling, wonton, or gyoza vegan wrappers

Dipping Sauce Ingredients:

4 tablespoons lime juice

½ cup tamari

1/8 cup rice vinegar

2 teaspoons red pepper flakes

Directions:

1. Add the diced mushrooms to large skillet and dry sauté for about 5 minutes, until softened. If too dry, add a little water to skillet.

2. Add the cabbage and the teaspoon of salt to the skillet.

3. Continue to cook, stirring occasionally, until the cabbage is completed wilted, 3-4 minutes. Transfer the mixture to a bowl and set aside until cool enough to handle.

4. Meanwhile, drain tofu in paper towels and then crumble into a large mixing bowl. Add the ginger, garlic, tamari, rice vinegar, and black pepper. Stir to combine.

5. Squeeze handfuls of the cooled mushroom-cabbage mixture to remove as much moisture as possible and transfer to the tofu mixture.

6. Stir to combine all the ingredients. Add more of any of the seasonings to taste.

7. Set a bowl of water and a baking sheet lined with parchment paper near your workspace.

8. Layer several dumpling wrappers on the work surface and place a scant tablespoon of filling in the middle of each. Dip a finger in the water and run it around the edge of the first dumpling wrapper.

9. Fold the wrapper over and pinch it closed. Repeat with the remaining wrappers until all the filling is used.

10. To cook the pot stickers, put in a steamer or bamboo steamer if you have one. Don't overfill steaming pan so water does not contact the dumplings.

11. Bring water to boil and steam the dumplings for 3-5 minutes, until the wrappers are translucent.

12. Serve immediately with dipping sauce.

SUSHI ROLLS

A Simple Guide created by Sherry Shrallow

Ingredients and Supplies:

Sushi rice (add rice vinegar, sugar and salt to taste)

Sushi rolling mat (can be found at any Asian grocery store)

Package of Nori (dried seaweed- also found at Asian grocery store or traditional stores)

Dried wasabi powder (follow directions on can to make)

Pickled ginger (in a jar is fine)

Chopsticks

Large plastic storage bag to place sushi mat into (for ease of cleaning)

Veggies of your choice - cut into 4 inch thin strips (I use cucumbers, carrots, cooked asparagus tips, roasted red peppers, and avocados.)

Directions:

1. Place sushi mat inside bag and squeeze out any excess air.

2. Place mat on flat surface. Take one sheet of Nori dried seaweed and cut in half. Place shiny side down. Lines should run horizontally as you place sheet onto your sushi mat.

3. Cover nori seaweed with cooked sushi rice, leaving a ½ inch area at the bottom of the sheet empty. You will need a bowl of water beside you to wet your hands so the rice will not stick to you.

4. Place 2-3 veggies in middle of roll running horizontally. Less is better in this case. Beginners often overstuff their rolls. Take your sushi mat and start rolling it towards you, pressing down gently on the mat as you roll up the nori seaweed over your veggies.

Take a little water and wet the ½ inch clear area of the nori seaweed at the bottom of your roll to close it. Continue to turn roll over and gently press down using your sushi mat to firm up the roll. This is called a Maki roll. You can also do an Inside Out sushi roll by flipping the nori seaweed with the rice covering the entire area before adding veggies and rolling. This way the rice will appear on the outside and you can even add some sesame seeds if you'd like on top of the rice.

5. Take a very sharp knife that you've wet with water and slice roll in half. Then slice the two halves again and you should have 4 nice sized sushi rolls. Dip into your prepared wasabi and soy sauce, and finish with a slice of pickled ginger to cool off your palette after eating rolls with the hot wasabi.

7 LAYER DIP

created By Andrew Olson at One Ingredient Chef

Ingredients:

One 15 -ounce can low fat refried or black beans

½ teaspoon coriander

½ teaspoon cayenne pepper

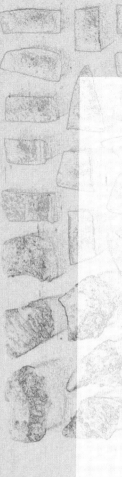

½ teaspoon cumin

1 avocado

1 lime, juiced

Pinch of salt

2/3 cup cashews, soaked for several hours

½ cup water

1 teaspoon apple cider vinegar

1 cup chopped romaine lettuce

¼ cup nutritional yeast

3 roma tomatoes

3 green onions

¼ cup chopped cilantro

¼ cup sliced olives (optional)

Directions:

1. Mix beans with spices. If using black beans, blend in food processor. Spoon this layer into bottom of glass dish.

2. In bowl, mash avocado, lime juice, and salt with a fork and spread layer over beans.

3. In blender, blend soaked cashews, apple cider vinegar, and water until smooth and resembles consistency of sour cream. Spread as layer three.

4. Chop lettuce and layer over cashew cream.

5. Seed tomatoes and dice. Spread evenly as next layer.

6. Make last layer with toppings of green onion, cilantro and olives. Serve spooned over corn tortilla chips.

EDAMAME WITH SPIKE SEASONING

created by Sherry Shrallow

I've cut out the salt to make this a healthier version

Ingredients:

½ teaspoon crushed red pepper flakes

1 tablespoon Spike seasoning

½ teaspoon sugar

1 pound frozen edamame in shells

Directions:

1. Pulse red pepper flakes in a grinder until finely ground. Mix with Spike seasoning and sugar in small bowl.

2. Bring a large pot of water to boil. Add frozen edamame and cook until bright green and heated through, about 4 minutes. Strain

and transfer to large bowl. Toss with the seasonings and serve.

COLLARD GREEN VEGGIE WRAPS WITH CREAMY PEANUT SAUCE

created by Terri Edwards

These collard green wraps offer a fresh, healthy appetizer that is bursting with vibrant color and loads of nutrition. The creamy peanut sauce can be made with peanut butter or PB2 for a lower-fat option You can also use the peanut sauce as a salad dressing.

Servings: 4 wraps

Wrap Ingredients:

4 whole collard green leaves

1 cup bulgur (this will be ½ cup of dry/uncooked)

1 cup carrots, grated

1 cup cucumber, sliced into strips

1 cup red bell pepper, sliced into strips

1 cup bean sprouts

½ cup peanut sauce (recipe below)

Peanut Sauce Recipe:

2 tablespoons Bragg Liquid Aminos or soy sauce

1 tablespoon rice vinegar or red wine vinegar

1 teaspoon minced garlic

3 tablespoons natural peanut butter or 6 tablespoons PB2 plus 3 tablespoons water

¼ cup almond milk (or more if needed to thin)

1 teaspoon Thai chili paste or ¼ teaspoon Sriracha sauce

Directions:

1. If needed, heat sauce ingredients in microwave for 30 seconds to allow for easier blending and set aside.

2. Collard greens are very large and rigid. Here's how to make them easier to work with. First, lay the collard leaf on a cutting board and turn it with the coarse side up. Use a sharp knife to trim the thickest part of the stem, being careful not to cut through the leaf. This will help the leaf to roll and be folded without cracking or tearing.

3. Bring a pot of water to a boil, then lower the heat to medium low. Hold the long stem of the leaf and dunk into the water for approximately 20-30 seconds, then quickly

remove leaf and lay it on cutting board or other flat surface. Each leaf will need to be dunked into the water separately.

4. Use scissors or a sharp knife to cut off long stem to level with the bottom of the leaf.

5. Begin by spooning 2-3 tablespoons of cooked bulgur onto the middle of the leaf, about ¼ of the way up the stem. Add all the other diced and grated vegetables and drizzle with approximately 2 tablespoons of the peanut sauce.

6. To roll, fold side edges of leaf over the middle filled portion. Fold the bottom (stem end) up and over the filling. Begin to roll up firmly to the end, then place the rolled side down on a plate. Serve immediately with the rest of the peanut sauce for dipping.

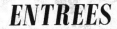

ENTREES

NEW OLD-FASHIONED TOFU LOAF

created by Mary McDougall from The Starch Solution

Ingredients:

30 ounces firm non-GMO tofu, drained well and mashed with a fork

1 2/3 cups quick-cooking oats (I used long cooking oats and it was fine)

¾ cup whole wheat bread crumbs (I used no-oil whole wheat panko bread crumbs)

½ cup ketchup or barbecue sauce

1/3 cup Bragg Liquid Aminos or low-sodium soy sauce

2 tablespoons dijon mustard

2 tablespoons vegetarian worcestershire sauce

¼ teaspoon garlic powder

¼ teaspoon freshly ground black pepper

Directions:

1. Preheat the oven to 350 degrees. Have on hand a nonstick standard or silicone loaf pan.

2. Put the tofu into a large bowl and add the remaining ingredients. Mix well with your hands until it is well combined.

3. Turn the mixture into your loaf pan and bake for about 1 hour, or until the top and edges are browned. Cool on rack for 5 minutes before serving.

TOFU LASAGNA

from Whole Foods Market

Ingredients:

One 14-ounce package firm non-GMO tofu, drained

2 tablespoons nutritional yeast

1 teaspoon garlic powder

Salt and pepper to taste

One 25-ounce jar fat free marinara sauce (Whole Foods, Engine 2 and Trader Joes have a fat-free version)

3 bell peppers, (red, yellow and orange combination is prettiest), cored, seeded and chopped

Fresh spinach, chopped or whole pieces (my addition)

12 no-boil whole grain dried lasagna noodles (I have used regular noodles that are not no boil and it works)

Directions:

1. Preheat oven to 350 degrees. Use a 9 x 13 baking dish- no need to use cooking spray.

2. Wrap tofu in 3 or 4 layers of paper towels and gently press out as much water as possible, changing the paper towels once or twice as needed. Transfer tofu to a large bowl and add nutritional yeast, garlic powder, salt and pepper and mash with a fork. Set tofu mixture aside.

3. Put marinara sauce and peppers into a medium pot, simmering until peppers are tender, about 10 minutes.

4. Spoon enough marinara sauce into baking dish to cover the bottom and then arrange 4 noodles on top. Spread 1/3 of the tofu mixture over the noodles, some fresh spinach on top of tofu mixture and then spread more sauce to cover. Repeat this process two

more times, ending with the sauce. I sprinkle nutritional yeast on top of sauce and then cover with foil and bake until noodles are tender, about one hour. Set aside to rest for 10 minutes and then serve.

5. Even better if you make ahead and reheat!

EGGPLANT BALLS

(contributor unknown)

Ingredients:

1 large eggplant, peeled and diced (See below Directions for how to prepare eggplant)

2 teaspoons onion, finely diced

2 cloves garlic, minced

1 cup Ian's Panko Bread Crumbs

2 teaspoons nutritional yeast

1 teaspoon oregano

½ teaspoon parsley flakes

¼ teaspoon salt

Ener-G Egg Replacer for 1 egg (or 1 tablespoon flaxseed mixed with 3 tablespoons water)

Directions:

1. Combine the panko bread crumbs, nutritional yeast, oregano, parsley and salt in a food processor. (I just mixed together in a large bowl). If processing, dump into large bowl.

2. In a large non-stick skillet, sauté the onion for about 5 minutes or until soft and translucent. Add the garlic and cook for another 5 minutes. Add to the breadcrumb mixture.

3. Using the same pan, sauté the eggplant for about 15 minutes or until soft and gray in color. Allow to cool.

4. Dump the eggplant into the food processor and process until smooth and sort of pasty. (I just kept mashing up the eggplant in the skillet until it was very mushy looking).

5. Add the egg replacer or the flaxseed and water mixture. Mix all together. Form balls using wet hands to avoid sticking and place on parchment lined baking sheet. Bake for 20-25 minutes at 375 degrees, flipping halfway through for even baking.

6. Make whole grain pasta or brown rice pasta and mix Eggplant balls into your favorite no-oil marinara sauce and serve over cooked pasta.

Preparing Eggplant:

Before getting started, drain the eggplant that is cut up for about an hour by placing it in a strainer with 1 teaspoon salt. Squeeze out the liquid in the eggplant after an hour before putting into skillet.

DOMINICAN BEANS

created by LeAnne Campbell in The China Study Cookbook

LeAnne prepared this meal for us when we went to her Global Roots Conference in the Dominican Republic. I don't think there was any left after we went at it. Delicious!

For The Beans

¼ cup vegetable broth, divided

1 onion, diced

4 cloves garlic, minced or pressed

1 medium green bell pepper, diced

½ cup diced butternut squash

½ cup chopped cilantro

1 cup water

3 tablespoons tomato paste

2 cans pinto, black or red beans

½ tablespoon Mexican oregano leaves, dried

½ teaspoon dried thyme

Sea salt to taste

4 cups cooked brown rice for serving

For The Salad

2 cups sliced lettuce

2 cups cabbage, sliced into strips

¾ cup sliced cucumber

¾ cup sliced cooked beets

1 tomato, sliced

1 large avocado, sliced

Balsamic rice vinegar

¼ teaspoon salt

¼ teaspoon pepper

Directions:

1. Heat 2 tablespoons vegetable broth in a large stock pot and sauté the onion and garlic over medium-high heat until soft. Add green pepper, squash, cilantro, and two more tablespoons vegetable broth. Cook for 2 minutes, stirring.

2. Add water, tomato paste, beans, oregano, and thyme. Bring to a simmer and cook,

uncovered, for 15 minutes. If needed, add an additional ½ cup water. Season with salt.

3. Make the salad in a large salad bowl. Serve beans over rice and top with salad.

SLOPPY LENTIL JOES

created by Ann Crile Esselstyn in
Prevent and Reverse Heart Disease

Ingredients:

3 1/3 cups water

1 large onion, chopped (1 cup)

1 bell pepper, any color-seeded and chopped (1 cup)

1 tablespoon chili powder

1 ½ cups dried lentils, red or brown

One 15 -ounce can salt-free crushed or diced tomatoes

1 tablespoon low-sodium tamari or Bragg Liquid Aminos

2 tablespoons mustard, dijon or your choice

1 tablespoon brown sugar (optional)

1 tablespoon rice vinegar

1 teaspoon vegan worcestershire sauce

1 bunch cilantro, chopped

Freshly ground black pepper, to taste

Directions:

1. Place 1/3 cup water in a large pot. Add onions and bell pepper and cook about 5 minutes, until onions soften slightly, stirring occasionally.

2. Add chili powder and mix well.

3. Add remaining water, the lentils, tomatoes, and the rest of the ingredients. Mix well, bring to a boil, lower heat, cover, and cook over low heat for 55 minutes, stirring occasionally.

4. Serve over brown rice or eat in a whole wheat bun.

SAUSAGE, PEPPER, AND MUSHROOM PIZZA

created by Chef Del Sroufe in The China Study Family Cookbook

Ingredients:

1 whole wheat pizza crust recipe (see recipe under Bread and Pizza Dough)

Cornmeal for dusting

1 to 1 ½ cups pizza sauce (see recipe under Sauces and Gravies)

½ recipe Spicy Breakfast Patties, crumbled (recipe below)

1 large yellow onion, diced

1 large green bell pepper, seeded and diced

8 ounces button mushrooms, sliced

Sea salt and black pepper

1 recipe Cheese Sauce (recipe below)

Chopped fresh basil, for garnish

Ingredients for Spicy Breakfast Patties:

Makes 14-16 patties

2 cups water

1 cup millet

¼ cup minced yellow onion

4 cloves garlic, minced

2 sun-dried tomatoes, minced

2 tablespoons tamari, or to taste

½ teaspoon dried sage

1 teaspoon crushed fennel seed

1 teaspoon crushed red pepper flakes, or to taste

¼ cup nutritional yeast

Sea salt

Instructions for Spicy Breakfast Patties:

1. Preheat oven to 350 degrees.

2. Combine the water and millet in a 2-quart saucepan with a tight-fitting lid. Bring to a boil over high heat. Reduce the heat to medium-low, cover the saucepan, and cook the millet until tender, about 20 minutes.

3. While the millet cooks, sauté the onion in a small skillet over medium-high heat until it turns translucent and starts to brown, about 5 minutes. Add water 1 or 2 tablespoons at a time to keep the onion from sticking to the pan.

4. Add the garlic, sun-dried tomatoes, tamari, sage, fennel, and red pepper flakes, and sauté for another minute to toast the seasonings. Remove the skillet from the heat. Add the nutritional yeast and cooked millet, season with sea salt to taste, and mix well.

5. Using a ¼ measuring cup or small ice cream scoop, shape the millet mixture into patties and place them on a baking sheet lined with parchment paper.

6. Bake for 15 minutes, turn over the patties, and continue to bake until the patties are firm to the touch and lightly browned, another 10 minutes or so. Serve warm.

Ingredients for the Cheese Sauce:

1 ½ cups finely diced russet potatoes (about 1 medium potato)

¼ cup finely diced red bell pepper

½ small yellow onion, diced

2 tablespoons raw cashews

2 tablespoons tahini

1 tablespoon fresh lemon juice

2 tablespoons nutritional yeast

2 tablespoons arrowroot powder

1 teaspoon sea salt, or to taste

Instructions for the Cheese Sauce:

1. Combine the potato, bell pepper, onion, and cashews in a small saucepan and cover with water. Bring the water to a boil over high heat. Reduce the heat to medium, and cook until the potatoes are very tender, about 10 minutes. Drain the vegetables, reserving ¾ cup of the cooking water.

2. Combine the potato mixture, reserved cooking water, tahini, lemon juice, nutritional yeast, arrowroot powder, and sea salt in a Vitamix blender. Process on high until everything is smooth and creamy, about 3 minutes. Store the sauce in an airtight container in the refrigerator for up to 5 days.

Instructions for Pizza Assembly:

1. Divide the pizza dough in half and shape each half into a round. Press the pizza dough onto each pizza pan or baking sheet. Spread half of the pizza sauce over each dough and distribute half of each of the toppings over the sauce.

2. Season with sea salt and black pepper to taste. Spoon the cheese sauce over the vegetables.

3. Bake until the crust is browned, 12 to 13 minutes. Remove pizza from the oven and garnish with the chopped basil.

SPINACH MUSHROOM QUICHE WITH POTATO CRUST

created by Kim Campbell at plantpurepods.com/recipes

Ingredients:

2 tablespoons flax meal or chia seeds

5 tablespoons water

2 large potatoes, shredded, rinsed and squeezed or one bag salt-free hash brown potatoes from Whole Foods or Trader Joes.

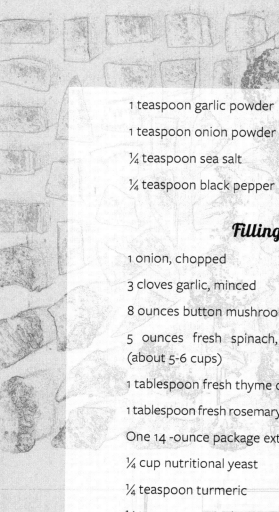

1 teaspoon garlic powder

1 teaspoon onion powder

¼ teaspoon sea salt

¼ teaspoon black pepper

Filling:

1 onion, chopped

3 cloves garlic, minced

8 ounces button mushrooms, sliced

5 ounces fresh spinach, roughly chopped (about 5-6 cups)

1 tablespoon fresh thyme or 1 teaspoon dried

1 tablespoon fresh rosemary or 1 teaspoon dried

One 14 -ounce package extra-firm tofu

¼ cup nutritional yeast

¼ teaspoon turmeric

½ teaspoon sea salt

¼ teaspoon black pepper

2 tomatoes, thinly sliced (optional, for topping)

Directions:

1. Preheat oven to 400 degrees. Line a 10-inch pie pan with parchment paper, cutting off excess paper around the edges.

2. In a small bowl, combine the flax meal or chia seeds with water. Set aside to thicken.

3. Peel and shred the potatoes if using fresh potatoes. Squeeze the moisture out of the potatoes and pat dry. Transfer to a bowl and add the flax mixture, garlic powder and onion powder. Mix thoroughly.

4. Pat the shredded potatoes into the prepared pie pan, making sure to cover the entire bottom and sides. Season with salt and pepper to taste. Bake for 10-15 minutes, until the potatoes begin to brown. Set aside to cool.

5. In a nonstick skillet over medium-high heat, sauté the onion, garlic, mushrooms, spinach, thyme, and rosemary in a small amount of water until tender, about 8 minutes. Remove from heat and drain any extra moisture from the vegetables.

6. Combine the tofu, nutritional yeast, salt and pepper in a food processor or blender and blend until smooth and creamy. Transfer to a mixing bowl and add the sautéed vegetables. Mix thoroughly.

7. Spread the tofu-mushroom mixture over the potato crust in the pie pan. Top with tomato slices if using.

8. Bake at 375 degrees for 30-40 minutes, or until firmly set. Let stand for 15-20 minutes, then cut into wedges to serve.

PASTA WITH VEGETABLES AND WHITE BEAN MISO SPREAD

created by Chef Del Sroufe in
The China Study Quick and Easy Cookbook

Serves 6

Ingredients:

1 pound whole grain penne pasta

One 12-ounce package frozen mixed vegetables (about 3 cups)

1 recipe White Bean-Miso Spread (recipe below)

Low-sodium vegetable stock to taste

1-2 teaspoons crushed red pepper flakes, to taste

8 green onions, thinly sliced

Instructions for White Bean-Miso Spread:

Add the following to a food processor and puree until smooth and creamy:

One 15-ounce can white beans (navy, great Northern, or cannellini), drained and rinsed

3 tablespoons mellow white miso paste

2 tablespoons almond butter (optional)

2 teaspoons granulated onion

½ teaspoon cayenne pepper (optional)

Instructions for Pasta with Vegetables and White Bean-Miso Spread:

1. Cook the pasta according to package instructions, adding the frozen vegetables to the pot with the pasta in the last 5 minutes of cooking.

2. While the pasta cooks, heat the White Bean Miso-Spread in a large saucepan over medium heat, stirring frequently. Thin the spread with a little vegetable stock to desired sauce consistency.

3. When the pasta and vegetables have finished cooking, drain them and add them to the sauce and mix well.

4. Serve garnished with red pepper flakes and the sliced green onions.

CAULIFLOWER FETTUCCINE ALFREDO WITH PINK PEPPERCORNS

created by Danielle Bussone in Time for Change and modified by Sherry Shrallow

Ingredients:

½ medium cauliflower, cut into florets (5 cups)

½ cup water

½ pound fettucine noodles

1 teaspoon chickpea miso

1 tablespoon nutritional yeast

¼ cup cashew cream cheese (recipe below)

¼ teaspoon whole pink peppercorns for garnish (or you can substitute a pinch of black pepper)

Salt to taste (optional)

CASHEW CREAM CHEESE

Ingredients:

1 ¼ cup cashews, soaked at least 5 hours or overnight.

1 tablespoon apple cider vinegar

Juice of 1-2 lemons (2 ½ -5 tablespoons)

¼ teaspoon salt

1-2 tablespoons freshly minced dill (optional)

Directions:

Add soaked and drained cashews to a high powered blender (I use a Vitamix), and add apple cider vinegar, lemon juice and salt. Blend until smooth. Transfer to a bowl and add minced dill. Chill for two hours in refrigerator for flavors to meld perfectly.

Directions for Fettuccine:

1. Cook pasta according to package instructions and drain.

2. Steam cauliflower in a saucepan in ½ cup water on medium-high heat until tender.

3. Add the cauliflower, cashew cream cheese, nutritional yeast, and miso into a blender and puree for about 2 minutes or until smooth. Add a little of the cauliflower water or filtered water to blender if it seems too thick.

4. Transfer to a medium saucepan. Heat through and adjust consistency by adding a little water if needed. Toss with fettucine noodles and top with a sprinkling of additional nutritional yeast.

"TURKEY" TETRAZZINI ALA SOY CURLS

*created by Debby Kastner, The Healthy Librarian and
adapted from Barb Watson's recipe and further adapted by
Sherry Shrallow*

Ingredients:

(8 generous servings 9 x 13 pan)

One 12-ounce package of brown rice spaghetti or any spaghetti of your choice.

2 cups of reconstituted Butler brand Soy Curls (1/2 of an 8-ounce package), drained and squeezed of excess liquid. Use a low sodium vegetable broth when soaking the curls for about 20 minutes.

Ingredients For Tetrazzini Sauce:

2 cups low-sodium vegetable broth

2 cups unsweetened soy milk

3 tablespoons cornstarch

½ cup raw cashews

1 medium onion, chopped

1 plus cup of celery chopped

8 ounces of white or cremini mushrooms, sliced

1 large portobello mushroom, sliced or chopped

Salt and freshly ground pepper to taste

½ teaspoon poultry seasoning, more if you like (it's vegan)

1/3-½ cup of sherry cooking wine

Directions:

Cook pasta per package directions. Set aside.

Preheat oven to 350 degrees.

Directions for the sauce:

1. Heat 2 cups of vegetable broth to almost a boil. Lower to medium heat.

2. In Vitamix, blend raw cashews with 1 cup of the soy milk and poultry seasoning until smooth and creamy. If you use a regular blender, you'll need to soak your cashews in water for about 4 hours and then rinse and drain before using.

3. Whisk cornstarch into 1 cup of unheated soy milk. Dissolve completely.

4. Add the cornstarch and unheated soy milk mixture into the almost boiling broth—whisking constantly, over medium heat, or until it starts to thicken and bubble just a bit—but, not a rolling boil. Once thickened add the blended cashew and soy milk into the broth soy milk mixture on the stove. Heat through until desired thickness. Adjust seasonings. Add the sherry.

Directions for cooking vegetables and soy curls:

1. In a large non-stick frying pan, sauté the onions, celery and mushrooms until they are softened and any liquid has evaporated. Covering the pan as they sauté keeps them from drying out. This takes about 7-10 minutes. Stir occasionally to keep from sticking. Add a little water if needed.

2. Add the rehydrated soy curls. Mix well. Season with fresh black pepper, salt and poultry seasoning.

3. Mix the spaghetti, sauce, vegetables and Soy Curls in a big bowl and combine.

4. Put mixture into 9 x 13 pan and top with ½ to 1 cup of Ian's panko bread crumbs of your choice. Cover with foil and bake for 20-30 minutes. Uncover and bake an additional 10-15 minutes, until it's bubbly and lightly browned.

THANKSGIVING MEATLESS LOAF

created by Susan Voisin at fatfreevegan.com

Ingredients:

1 medium sweet potato

1 medium onion

2 ribs celery

1 medium carrot

2 cloves garlic, minced

One 15 -ounce can cannellini beans, drained and rinsed

One 14 -ounce extra firm tofu

2 tablespoons Bragg Liquid Aminos

2 tablespoons tomato paste

1 tablespoon spicy brown mustard or whole-grain mustard

¼ cup fresh parsley, chopped

½ tablespoon rubbed sage

1 tablespoon thyme leaf

½ tablespoon dried rosemary, crushed

1 ½ teaspoons salt

½ teaspoon black pepper

1 teaspoon smoked paprika

2 tablespoons nutritional yeast

½ cup chopped walnuts, optional

¾ cup quinoa flakes

Directions:

1. Bake, steam or microwave sweet potato until soft. Mince the onion, celery, and carrot until finely chopped. Food processor makes it easier if you have one. Heat a large non-stick skillet and add the minced vegetables, including the garlic, and cook until tender, stirring for about 6-10 minutes. Add water by the teaspoon to avoid sticking. Add the drained beans and mash them lightly with a slotted spoon or spatula.

2. Place the peeled and cooked sweet potato into a food processor along with the tofu, Braggs, and all the seasonings. Process until fairly smooth. Add the walnuts and pulse a few more times. Scrape the tofu mixture into a large bowl and add the quinoa flakes and the cooked vegetables. Stir well.

3. Preheat oven to 375 degrees. Line a baking sheet with parchment paper and shape the tofu mixture into a loaf form 2 ½ inches high on the parchment paper using dampened hands. Bake 25 minutes or until the top is evenly browned. Loosely cover with parchment paper and cook for 20

more minutes. Check to make sure that the center is firm. If not, cook a little longer. For a crunchier crust, remove the parchment paper at end for 5 more minutes. Remove from oven and allow to stand for 10 minutes before slicing and serving. (Delicious covered with mushroom gravy.)

BBQ SOY CURLS

created by Leslie Haas and adapted from Carol Korbutt's Soy Curl and BBQ recipe

Ingredients:

One 8-ounce bag of Butler Soy Curls

16-ounce jar of barbecue sauce

8 ounces low sodium fat free vegetable broth

8 ounces very warm water

½ large onion, diced, preferably a vidalia onion

2 teaspoons black pepper

2 teaspoons poultry seasoning or Spike seasoning

Directions:

1. Place soy curls into a medium sized bowl.
2. Pour vegetable broth and very warm water

over the Soy Curls.

3. If needed, add more warm water until the curls are covered and then soak for 10 minutes.

4. Sauté onion in fry pan or Instant pot until they glisten.

5. After Soy Curls have soaked for 10 minutes, squeeze out excess moisture a handful at a time and place in your sauté pan. Sprinkle with poultry seasoning, pepper and barbecue sauce.

6. Heat on medium heat until edges begin to darken a little, and then remove from heat.

7. Serve on open toasted buns such as Ezekiel brand, which are oil-free.

CURRIED POTATOES WITH CHICKPEAS

created by Kim Campbell in The PlantPure Nation Cookbook

Ingredients:

4 potatoes, peeled and cubed

1 onion, diced

3 garlic cloves, minced

2 teaspoons ground cumin

¼ teaspoon cayenne pepper

1 tablespoon Thai Kitchen Red Curry Paste

4 teaspoons garam masala (recipe below), or just buy this seasoning at the store

1 teaspoon grated fresh ginger

1 teaspoon sea salt

One 14-ounce can diced tomatoes

One 15-ounce can chickpeas, rinsed and drained

1 ½ cups frozen peas

2/3 cup lite coconut milk

Directions:

1. Place the potatoes into a large pot and cover with water. Bring to a boil over high heat, then reduce the heat to medium-low, cover, and simmer until just tender, 10-15 minutes. Be careful not to overcook the potatoes and create a mushy texture.

2. Drain the potatoes and set aside.

3. Sauté the onion and garlic in a little water until tender, about 5 minutes. Season with the cumin, cayenne, curry paste, garam masala, ginger, and salt. Cook for 2 minutes more.

4. Add the tomatoes, chickpeas, frozen peas and cooked potatoes.

5.   Pour in the coconut milk and bring to a simmer for 5-10 minutes.

GARAM MASALA

This spice blend is used in many Indian dishes.

Ingredients:

1 tablespoon ground cumin

1 ½ teaspoons ground coriander

1 ½ teaspoons ground cardamom

1 ½ teaspoons black pepper

1 teaspoon ground cinnamon

½ teaspoon ground cloves

½ teaspoon ground nutmeg

1 teaspoon ground ginger

Directions:

Mix all the ingredients and store in an airtight container in a cool, dry place

PALAK PANEER, TOFU STYLE

created by Kim Campbell in The PlantPure Nation Cookbook

Ingredients:

One 14-ounce block extra firm tofu, cut into ½ inch cubes

One 13-ounce can lite coconut milk

1 teaspoon sea salt, divided

1 large onion, diced

6 garlic cloves, minced

1 tablespoon finely grated ginger

1 ¼ cups water, divided

¼ teaspoon ground turmeric

1 teaspoon garam masala

1 teaspoon curry powder

1/8 teaspoon ground cloves

1 teaspoon whole fennel seeds

1-2 jalapeño peppers, seeded and minced

One 14-ounce can diced tomatoes

1 pound, chopped frozen spinach

4 cups cooked brown rice or naan bread for serving

3 tablespoons chopped cilantro, for garnish

Directions:

1. Preheat oven to 375 degrees. Line a baking sheet with parchment paper and set aside.

2. In a bowl, toss the cubed tofu in the coconut milk and ½ teaspoon sea salt and let marinate for 1 hour.

3. Strain the tofu from the coconut milk, reserving the coconut milk. Spread the tofu on the prepared baking sheet and bake for 20-25 minutes, tossing every 5-10 minutes.

4. Place the onion, garlic, and ginger in a food processor and grind into a paste. Transfer the paste to a medium-size pot with ¼ cup of the water and cook over medium heat for about 10 minutes, allowing the mixture to slightly caramelize.

5. Turn the heat down to low and add the turmeric, garam masala, curry powder, cloves, fennel seeds, and jalapeno (use 2 if you like it spicier). Simmer for 1-2 minutes. Add the tomatoes and stir to combine.

6. In a separate pan, steam the spinach over medium heat with the remaining 1 cup water until completely heated through.

7. Transfer the spinach to a food processor and puree until smooth. Transfer to the pot with the tomatoes and spices.

8. Allow this mixture to simmer over low heat

while your tofu finishes baking. Add the remaining ½ teaspoon sea salt and stir.

9.   When the tofu finishes baking, add it to the spinach mixture along with the reserved coconut milk from the tofu marinade.

10. Serve over rice, garnished with the cilantro.

SHERRY'S EASY BREEZY VEGETABLE AND TOFU STIR FRY

This recipe is quick and easy and can be done in 30 minutes.

Ingredients:

1 head of broccoli, chopped into small pieces

3 scallions, cut into small pieces

2 carrots, grated and cut into thin pieces along a diagonal

1 large red pepper, cut into 1-inch pieces

8 ounces mushrooms, sliced

One package extra firm non-GMO tofu, cut into one inch cubes

Any other vegetable you would like in your stir fry

One 9.7 ounce bottle of Annie Chun's Shitake

Soy Ginger sauce (found at Whole Foods). Low in sodium and oil-free!

Directions:

1. In a large fry pan, sauté all the stir fry vegetables with a little water until crisp tender. Toss in the tofu cubes, cover with stir fry sauce and heat thoroughly.

2. Serve over brown rice or brown rice noodles.

BURGERS, SANDWICHES AND WRAPS

UNFRIED FALAFELS

from Healthy Girl's Kitchen

Serves 8

Ingredients:

2-3 large cloves garlic

Packed ½ cup fresh flat leaf (Italian) parsley

Packed ½ cup fresh cilantro

½ cup scallions, rough chopped

Two 15 -ounce cans chickpeas, rinsed and drained-reserving at least 2 tablespoons of the liquid

1 cup rolled oats

1 ½ tablespoons fresh lemon juice

2 teaspoons ground cumin

1 teaspoon ground turmeric

1 ½ teaspoons ground coriander

1 teaspoon salt (omit if wanting low sodium)

¼ teaspoon pepper

¼-½ teaspoon crushed red pepper flakes

Directions:

1. Place garlic, parsley, cilantro, and scallions in the bowl of a food processor and process until mixture is finely chopped.

2. Add all other ingredients and process, scraping down the sides as necessary, until all ingredients are blended, but do not over process into a paste. You want the mixture to have a bit of its texture left, but be able to stick together easily. If mixture is too dry, add the reserved liquid from the chickpeas, one tablespoon at a time, pulsing to incorporate the liquid.

3. Transfer the mixture into a bowl and refrigerate for 30 minutes.

4. Form into patties and place one at a time onto a nonstick skillet that has been pre-heated over medium-high heat. Cook 5 minutes and then flip patties and cook another 5 minutes. Patties should be nicely browned and crisp but not burned.

5. Serve in pita bread and top with a tzatziki sauce (See tzatziki sauce recipe under Sauces and Gravies)

EASY BLACK BEAN BURGER

created by Kim Campbell in The PlantPure Nation Cookbook

Ingredients:

1 tablespoon flaxseed meal

3 tablespoons water

2 cans of black beans, rinsed and drained

½ cup cooked brown rice

¾ cups frozen corn

½ cup finely chopped onion

1 teaspoon cumin

½ teaspoon salt

1 teaspoon Mexican seasoning

3 tablespoons salsa

Directions:

1. Mix the flaxseed with water and set aside

2. In a large bowl, mash black beans with a fork, leaving some partially mashed. Add rice, corn, onion, cumin, salt, Mexican seasoning, salsa and flaxseed mixture and combine.

3. Shape into patties and place on parchment lined baking sheet.

4. Bake at 375 degrees in oven for 25 minutes.

Serve with your favorite condiments on an oil-free bun.

TOFU BURGERS

(creator unknown)

Ingredients:

14 ounces firm non-GMO tofu, drained

¼ cup whole grain flour (or use gluten free)

¼ cup cornmeal

1/3 cup rolled oats (or use gluten free)

1 cup fresh chopped parsley

1 teaspoon dried basil

1 teaspoon paprika (I used smoked paprika)

1 teaspoon dried coriander

½ teaspoon dried thyme

½ teaspoon dried ginger

¼ teaspoon salt

½ teaspoon garlic powder

½ teaspoon onion powder

½ teaspoon pepper

1 tablespoon Bragg Liquid Aminos (or low sodium soy sauce)

Directions:

1. Mash tofu with a fork in large mixing bowl and add rest of ingredients. I add a little water to mixture as it helps hold the burgers together.

2. Shape into patties and bake on a parchment paper lined baking sheet at 350 degrees for 30 minutes. I also put a dot of catsup in the middle of each burger.

EDAMAME BURGER

created by Kim Campbell in The PlantPure Nation Cookbook

Ingredients:

4 cups frozen shelled edamame, cooked

2 cups frozen mixed Asian vegetable stir-fry, thawed

1 tablespoon flax meal

2 tablespoons water

¼ cup orange juice

¼ teaspoon low-sodium soy sauce

1 tablespoon maple syrup or agave nectar

¼ teaspoon dijon mustard

1 cup whole wheat bread crumbs (I use Ian's Panko Bread Crumbs)

½ teaspoon sea salt

¼ teaspoon black pepper

1 teaspoon lemon juice

6 whole wheat oil-free burger buns

6 green-leaf lettuce leaves

1 ½ cups sprouts

¾ cup Cilantro-Wasabi Aioli (recipe below)

Directions:

1. Preheat oven to 375 degrees. Line a baking sheet with parchment paper.

2. Place the cooked edamame and thawed stir-fry blend into a food processor. Pulse multiple times until the ingredients are well blended. It should be green and have a fine consistency like that of short-grain rice.

3. In a small bowl, combine the flax meal and water. Allow to sit for 2-3 minutes.

4. Remove the vegetable mixture from the food processor and place in a large mixing bowl. Add the flax mixture and fold together.

5. Add the orange juice, soy sauce, maple syrup, dijon mustard, bread crumbs, salt, pepper and lemon juice to the vegetables and mix well.

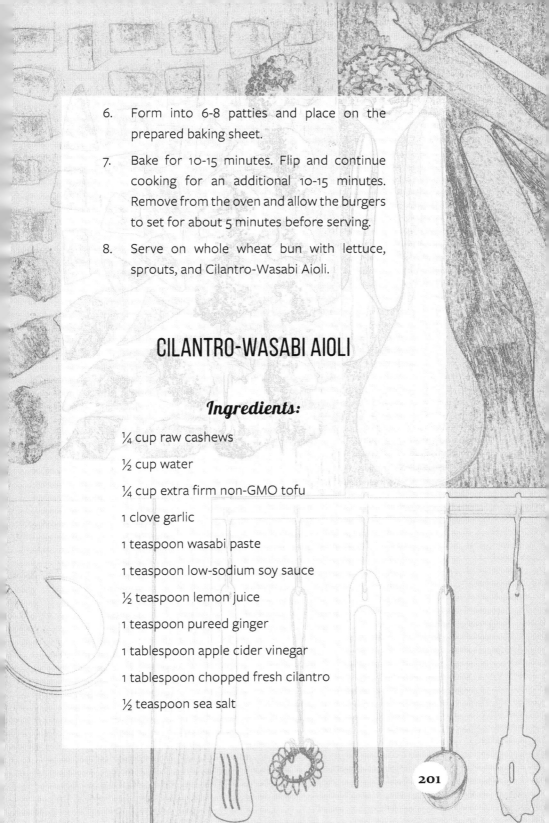

6. Form into 6-8 patties and place on the prepared baking sheet.

7. Bake for 10-15 minutes. Flip and continue cooking for an additional 10-15 minutes. Remove from the oven and allow the burgers to set for about 5 minutes before serving.

8. Serve on whole wheat bun with lettuce, sprouts, and Cilantro-Wasabi Aioli.

CILANTRO-WASABI AIOLI

Ingredients:

¼ cup raw cashews

½ cup water

¼ cup extra firm non-GMO tofu

1 clove garlic

1 teaspoon wasabi paste

1 teaspoon low-sodium soy sauce

½ teaspoon lemon juice

1 teaspoon pureed ginger

1 tablespoon apple cider vinegar

1 tablespoon chopped fresh cilantro

½ teaspoon sea salt

Directions:

1. Combine all the ingredients in a Vitamix or other high-powered blender and process on high speed until smooth and creamy.

2. Remove from the blender and chill to thicken. Serve chilled.

SHERRY'S FAVORITE WRAP

This wrap is my favorite quick go to lunch that I often take to work. Can be put together in minutes. Use your imagination and create your own favorite wrap with whatever ingredients you like. Here are some that I love to use.

Ingredients:

Oil-free hummus of your choice

Spinach, kale or lettuce (or a combination of greens)

Tomato slice

Sliced red pepper

Sprouts

Pita bread made without oil

Directions:

1. Slather your favorite hummus in the pita bread.

2. Stuff with remaining ingredients.

KALE AND SAUERKRAUT SANDWICH

created by Ann Crile Esselstyn and Jane Esselstyn in The Prevent and Reverse Heart Disease Cookbook

Hint: Use horseradish that is lower in sodium, such as Eden Organic or Bubbies, and rinse before using. Ann Esselstyn loves to make this with the Engine 2 Jalapeno Cilantro Hummus along with a horseradish mustard. The beauty of this sandwich is that you can vary your hummus selection to have a different tasting sandwich each time you make it.

Ingredients:

4 slices whole-grain bread

4 tablespoons Our Hummus (recipe found under Appetizer recipes section)

3-4 tablespoons prepared horseradish mustard or other mustard of your choice

1 bunch cooked kale or greens of your choice

½ cup prepared sauerkraut, rinsed and drained

8 cherry tomatoes, halved, or 1 small tomato, sliced

Directions:

1. Preheat a panini press. (If you don't have one, preheat a non-stick griddle and place a heavy pot on top of sandwich while cooking to get the "pressed" effect.)

2. Lay the slices of bread in pairs. Spread one slice of each pairing with the hummus and the other slice with the mustard.

3. Squeeze any extra liquid out of the kale with your hands. Do the same with the sauerkraut. You don't want soggy bread.

4. Spread a layer of kale on top of the hummus, then spread a layer of sauerkraut on top of the kale, and tomatoes on top of the sauerkraut. Place the mustard-covered bread on top, mustard side down.

5. Heat the sandwiches on both sides until nicely browned and warmed through. Cut on an angle and serve.

SIDE DISHES

CRISPY OVEN BAKED FRIES

created by Susan Voisin at fatfreevegan.com

Ingredients:

7-8 small to medium sized potatoes

1 tablespoon whole wheat flour

1 teaspoon garlic powder

1 teaspoon onion powder

1 teaspoon paprika

1 teaspoon chili powder

Spike seasoning to taste

Directions:

1. Preheat oven to 425 degrees.

2. Line a large cookie sheet with parchment paper.

3. Clean and slice potatoes with skin on into thick french fries

4. Add to a pot of cold water and cover. Bring to a boil.

5. Boil for 5 minutes.

6. After boiling, drain potatoes and put back into pot. Add all seasonings and shake to distribute.

7. Spread evenly on cookie sheet lined with parchment paper and bake for 20-25 minutes.

SHERRY'S MARVELOUS MASHED POTATOES

I created these mashed potatoes by tasting as I went along. Adjust seasonings to your liking and add new ones to create your very own mashed potato recipe.

Ingredients:

4 large red potatoes

½ cup non-dairy unsweetened milk of your choice

1 teaspoon garlic powder

1 teaspoon onion powder

Spike seasoning and pepper to taste

Directions:

1. Rinse potatoes and dice into quarters. Place into pot of boiling water and boil for about 15-20 minutes, or until tender.

2. Drain potatoes and place into large mixing bowl. Add rest of ingredients and mash with a potato masher or with an electric mixer.

3. Serve with gravy of your choice.

MAPLE MASHED SWEET POTATOES

created by Mary McDougall in The McDougall Newsletter October 2005 Vol. 4 No. 10

I make every Thanksgiving and many other times throughout the year. Simple to make and oh so delicious.

Serves 6

Ingredients:

3 pounds sweet potatoes

½ cup unsweetened soy milk (or any non-dairy milk of your choice)

1 tablespoon pure maple syrup

Dash of salt (I omit)

Freshly ground pepper to taste

Directions:

1. You can bake or boil the sweet potatoes. I usually peel them and boil them as it is a

lot faster. Drain off cooking water before adding other ingredients to begin mashing.

2. If baking, scrub potatoes and prick all over with a fork. Place on a baking sheet and bake for about 45 minutes, or until potatoes are tender. Remove from oven and allow to cool slightly. Cut potatoes in half lengthwise and scoop out the flesh into a large bowl. Mash with a hand masher or electric beater. Add milk, maple syrup, and seasonings. Mix well.

"CREAMED" KALE

from WholeFoodsMarket.com

My daughter sent me this recipe back in 2011 and I've been loving it ever since.

Serves 4

Ingredients:

½ cup low-sodium vegetable broth

1 white onion, finely chopped

1 cup unsweetened soy milk or any other non-dairy milk

¼ cup raw cashews

2 tablespoons nutritional yeast

1 teaspoon onion powder

1 teaspoon mellow white miso (or chickpea miso)

Pinch of freshly grated nutmeg (or a pinch of dry nutmeg)

Pinch of red pepper flakes

4 cups chopped kale or other dark, leafy green

Directions:

1. Heat broth in a large skillet over medium heat. Add onion and cook until softened, 5 to 7 minutes. Transfer to a Vitamix blender or food processor, add milk, cashews, nutritional yeast, onion powder, miso, nutmeg and pepper flakes and puree until smooth.

2. Transfer blended mixture back to skillet and bring to a simmer over medium heat. Stir in kale and continue simmering, tossing until kale is just tender, about 5 minutes.

BRUSSELS SPROUTS WITH APPLES AND SHALLOTS

from WholeFoodsMarket.com

Serves 4 to 6

Ingredients:

1 pound brussels sprouts

2 large shallots, sliced into ¼ inch thick rings

2 medium crisp, firm apples (such as Gala, Honeycrisp or Braeburn), cored and cut into ½ inch chunks

½ cup water, divided

¼ cup apple cider vinegar, divided

¼ teaspoon sea salt

½ teaspoon freshly ground black pepper

4 sprigs fresh thyme

Directions:

1. Rinse brussels sprouts well and pull off any loose or yellowing leaves. Trim the stem ends and then quarter each sprout. Set aside.

2. Heat a large high-sided sauté pan over high heat. Add shallots to the very hot pan and cook, stirring constantly for 2 minutes. Add

apples and ¼ cup water, scraping any brown bits from the bottom as the water sizzles. Cook until the liquid reduces by half, about 2 minutes. Add brussels sprouts, remaining ¼ cup water, 2 tablespoons apple cider vinegar, salt and pepper. Reduce heat to medium, cover and simmer until the sprouts and apples are tender enough to be pierced all the way through with a fork, stirring occasionally, about 15 minutes.

3. Uncover, stir in remaining 2 tablespoons of apple cider vinegar and the leaves pulled from sprigs of thyme. Scrape any bits from the bottom of the pan as liquid sizzles and reduces until nearly gone. Transfer to a serving bowl with any of the remaining liquid and serve immediately.

LOUBIEH BRAISED GREEN BEANS

created by Wendy Solganik at Healthy Girls Kitchen

Serves 6

Ingredients:

2 cups yellow onions, diced

2 cloves garlic, minced

One 15-ounce can diced tomatoes with juice

1 pound fresh green beans, ends trimmed off
and cut into thirds

½ cup water

1 tablespoon maple syrup

Salt and pepper to taste

Directions:

1. Dry sauté onions for about 20 minutes. Add small amounts of water to avoid sticking.

2. Add garlic and continue sautéing for an additional 3-4 minutes. Add tomatoes and juice and cook for 3 more minutes. Add green beans, maple syrup and water and cover.

3. Reduce heat to medium low and cook for 45 minutes. Season with salt and pepper to taste.

SAUCES AND GRAVIES

SWEET & SOUR SAUCE

created by Josh Latham from myvegancookbook.com

I use this sauce to dip my zucchini fritters into.

Ingredients:

One 8-ounce can pineapple chunks

¼ cup sugar

1 tablespoon Black Strap Molasses

¼ cup rice vinegar

1 teaspoon paprika

2 teaspoons corn starch

½ teaspoon salt

Directions:

Blend all ingredients in a Vitamix or immersion blender until smooth. Pour into a saucepan and cook on medium high heat, stirring constantly until sauce thickens.

DELICIOUS EASY HOMEMADE PIZZA SAUCE

contributed by Brandi Doming at TheVegan8.com

Ingredients:

2 cups tomato puree

1 teaspoon onion powder

1 teaspoon garlic powder

1 ½ teaspoons dried oregano

1 ½ teaspoons dried basil

½ teaspoon dried thyme

¼ teaspoon ground black pepper

1 tablespoon pure maple syrup

½ teaspoon fine sea salt (if your tomato puree is salt-free, you may need to add a little more)

½ teaspoon crushed red pepper flakes

Directions:

Add all the ingredients to a bowl and stir until well combined. Is best if you can store in refrigerator overnight but can use right away if needed.

RED LENTIL MARINARA SAUCE

created by Karen Kornick

Ingredients:

1 large onion

8 ounces portabella mushrooms, diced

10 ounces fresh spinach

3 cloves minced garlic

½ teaspoon dried thyme

½ teaspoon dried oregano

Salt and pepper to taste

One 28-ounce can salt-free whole peeled tomatoes (San Marzano preferably)

2 tablespoons tomato paste

2 cups vegetable broth

1 teaspoon honey (can substitute agave nectar)

1 cup red lentils

Fresh basil leaves (10 leaves)

Directions:

1. In a large pot, add onions, spinach and mushrooms and cook, stirring occasionally until soft, about 5 minutes, adding water as

needed to avoid sticking. Add the remaining ingredients (except the basil leaves) and stir to incorporate. Heat until the mixture comes to a boil and then reduce heat to medium-low. Simmer sauce for about 25 minutes or until the lentils are tender.

2. Stir in basil. Taste and add additional salt or pepper if desired.

3. Serve with your favorite whole grain pasta.

4. Can be kept in refrigerator 3-4 days or freeze for up to 3 months.

THAI DIPPING SAUCE

creator unknown

Ingredients:

¾ cup water

2 teaspoons cornstarch

1/3 cup seasoned rice vinegar

¼ cup brown sugar

1 ½ tablespoons reduced sodium soy sauce or Bragg Liquid Aminos

1 tablespoon fresh ginger, grated (or ginger found in jar in produce refrigerated section)

2 cloves garlic, mashed

½ teaspoon crushed red pepper flakes

Directions:

1. Whisk together all the ingredients in a small saucepan.

2. Bring to a boil, waiting until it thickens.

3. Cool to room temperature.

TZATZIKI SAUCE FOR FALAFELS

from Family Life in the Hollars

Ingredients:

6-8 ounces of plain soy yogurt

1 cucumber, peeled and seeded and chopped into small pieces

Juice from ½ lemon

3 tablespoons dill weed

1-2 cloves garlic, minced

Salt and pepper to taste

Directions:

Blend all ingredients into a bowl and chill until ready to serve

EASY MUSHROOM GRAVY

created by Ann Crile Esselstyn in Prevent and Reverse Heart Disease

Ingredients:

1 onion, chopped

2-3 garlic cloves, minced

One 10-ounce box mushrooms, sliced

Vegetable broth, wine, or water

2 cups water

2 tablespoons whole wheat flour

1 tablespoon miso, or Bragg Liquid Aminos

2 tablespoons sherry (optional)

Black pepper

Directions:

1. Stir-fry onion in a heavy saucepan over medium heat, adding water or broth as necessary. Allow onion to brown a little, scape the pan, add liquid, and let it brown more, but watch carefully so it does not burn. Add garlic and sliced mushrooms and continue cooking until mushrooms are soft. Add vegetable broth, wine, or water as necessary to keep from burning.

2. Add 1 cup of water (or vegetable broth for more intense flavor), stir, and continue cooking.

3. Mix whole-wheat flour and Bragg Liquid Aminos (or miso) in the remaining cup of water, stir, then add to the mushrooms and stir again. Add sherry (optional).

4. Continue cooking until gravy thickens. Add pepper to taste. Add extra miso or Braggs to taste if needed. Keep warm over low heat until serving.

NO COOK INSTANT BLENDER GRAVY

created by Anja Cass from cookingwithplants.com

Ingredients:

One 15-ounce can of chickpeas, drained and rinsed

½ cup nutritional yeast

¼ cup scallions, sliced

2 tablespoons miso paste (soy or chickpea)

2 tablespoons tamari, low-sodium soy sauce or Bragg Liquid Aminos

¼ teaspoon white pepper

1 large clove garlic, peeled

1 teaspoon dried sage leaves

1-2 cups hot boiled water

Directions:

Place all the ingredients into a blender and blend until smooth (about 1 minute)

CAULIFLOWER ALFREDO SAUCE

created by Kim Campbell in The PlantPure Nation Cookbook

Ingredients:

1 cauliflower head, broken into florets

½ teaspoon garlic powder

1 teaspoon onion powder

2 cups nondairy milk

¼ cup nutritional yeast flakes

1 tablespoon dijon mustard

½ teaspoon sea salt

½ teaspoon black pepper

Directions:

1. Bring a large pot of water to a boil and add

the cauliflower florets. Boil for about 15 minutes, or until tender.

2. Strain the cauliflower and add to a Vitamix or other blender with the remaining ingredients. Add nondairy milk for a thinner or thicker consistency. Blend until smooth and creamy.

CRANBERRY SAUCE

creator unknown

Ingredients:

2 cups fresh or frozen cranberries

1 ripe pear, peeled and diced

½ cup maple syrup

Pinch of fine sea salt

Directions:

Add cranberries, pear, maple syrup and salt to a pot and bring to a boil. Reduce heat to medium high and simmer uncovered for 10-20 minutes.

BREADS AND PIZZA DOUGH

WHOLE WHEAT PIZZA CRUST

created by Chef Del Sroufe in The China Study Family Cookbook

Makes 2 (12inch) pizzas

Ingredients:

One ¼ ounce packet active dry yeast

1 tablespoon cane sugar, such as sucanat

1 cup warm water (about 110 degrees)

½ teaspoon sea salt

About 2 cups whole wheat bread flour, divided

Directions:

1. In a large bowl, whisk together the yeast, sugar, and warm water. Let the mixture sit until it starts to foam, then add the sea salt, and, using a whisk, stir in 1 cup of the flour.

2. Beat the dough for 75 strokes. Add as much of the remaining 1 cup flour as needed to make a dough that is stiff but still a little tacky to the touch.

3. Cover the dough with plastic wrap and let

it sit in a warm place until it has doubled in volume, about 45 minutes. Punch it down and let it rise again, about 20 minutes.

4. Divide the dough in half and shape each half into a round. Press the pizza dough onto a pizza pan dusted with cornmeal, cover with homemade pizza sauce and your favorite veggie toppings and bake at 425 degrees for 12 to 13 minutes.

NAAN BREAD

created by Kim Campbell in The PlantPure Nation Cookbook

Use this bread to dip into your Curried Potatoes or Palak Paneer, Tofu Style (found under Entrees section)

Yields: 18-20 pieces

Ingredients:

1 tablespoon active dry yeast

1 cup warm water

1/3 cup agave nectar

¾ cup unsweetened soy milk

2 ¼ teaspoons Ener-G Egg Replacer mixed with 1 tablespoon water

½ teaspoon garlic powder

1 teaspoon rice vinegar

1 ½ teaspoons sea salt

4 cups whole wheat flour, as needed.

Directions:

1. In a large bowl, dissolve the yeast in the warm water. Let stand until frothy.

2. Stir in the agave, soy milk, egg replacer mixture, garlic powder, vinegar, salt and flour to make a soft dough. You may have to add flour depending on the type of flour you use. Do NOT use pastry flour because it will produce a gummy dough.

3. Turn out onto a lightly floured surface and knead for 6-8 minutes until smooth. Place the dough in a bowl and cover with a damp towel. Set aside in a warm place to rise until doubled in size, about 1 hour.

4. Punch down the dough and then pinch the dough into 18-20 small nectarine size balls. Place on a dry tray and allow to double in size, about 30 minutes.

5. Preheat a griddle pan over medium-high heat. On a work surface, next to the griddle, roll out one of the dough balls and stretch out the dough to form an uneven roundish shape.

6. Place on the griddle. Cook for 2-3 minutes, until puffy and lightly golden. Do not overcook; you want them to be able to fold without cracking. Turn over and cook the other side.

7. Continue to make all the naan until finished. Naan bread freezes well.

PHILLY-STYLE SOFT PRETZELS

created by Ann Crile Esselstyn and Jane Esselstyn in The Prevent and Reverse Heart Disease Cookbook

Ingredients:

¾ cup warm water

One (1 ¼ ounce) packet active dry yeast

2 tablespoons maple syrup

2 cups white whole wheat flour, plus more for kneading

½ cup oat flour

2 tablespoons baking soda

Topping of choice—a sprinkle of whatever you choose: nutritional yeast, poppy seeds, onion flakes, caraway seeds, kosher salt, pepper, or sesame seeds

Directions:

1. In a large bowl, mix together the warm water, yeast, maple syrup, and flours. Stir until the dough forms a large clump with an elastic feel.

2. Divide the dough into 6 equal clumps—each about the size of a small egg—and form them into balls. Place them back in the bowl. Cover the bowl with a damp kitchen towel and let the dough balls rise for at least 25 minutes.

3. Preheat the oven to 400 degrees. Line a baking sheet with parchment paper.

4. Bring a large pot of water to a boil and add the baking soda.

5. On a lightly floured surface, knead each dough ball, then roll it out into a rope, 12 to 18 inches long. Form a pretzel shape or any other shape you wish. Set the raw pretzel onto a slotted spoon and place it into the boiling water for 10 seconds. Remove the pretzel from the water with the slotted spoon and place it onto the lined baking sheet. While still damp, sprinkle or coat the pretzel with toppings of choice, or nothing at all.

6. Repeat for the other balls of dough.

7. When all the pretzels have been boiled, and topped, bake for 12 to 15 minutes.

8. These are best when served hot.

DESSERTS

KIM'S CHICK PEA CHOCLATE CHIP DELIGHTS

created by Kim Campbell at Plantpurenation.com,

Ingredients:

1 tablespoon flax meal or chia seeds

3 tablespoons water

1 ½ cups oats

½ cup powdered peanut butter (I use PB2) *see alternative below

¾ teaspoon baking powder

¾ teaspoon baking soda

¼ teaspoon sea salt

1 cup vegan chocolate chips

One 15-ounce can garbanzo beans, drained and rinsed

¾ cup plant-based milk

¾ cup sucanat

2 teaspoons vanilla

Directions:

1. Preheat oven to 375 degrees. Line a baking sheet with parchment paper.

2. In a small bowl, mix the flax meal (or chia seeds) with the water and set aside to thicken.

3. In a blender or food processor, process the oats into flour. Transfer to a large mixing bowl and add the powdered peanut butter, baking powder, baking soda, salt, and chocolate chips. Mix until thoroughly combined.

4. In the same blender (no need to rinse out), combine the chickpeas, milk, sucanat, and vanilla. Blend until very smooth and creamy.

5. Fold the chickpea mixture into the dry ingredient mixture and mix only until combined. Fold in the flaxseed or chia with water as well. Do not overmix.

6. Drop spoonful of the cookie dough onto the prepared baking sheet. I like to shape my cookies by dipping a spoon into water, then smoothing out each cookie and pressing down slightly to flatten them. This keeps them uniform and smooth. Baked for 10-12 minutes, until dry and lightly golden.

*If you can't find PB2 powdered peanut butter use 1/3 cup all-natural peanut butter and reduce the milk to ½ cup. This will add to the fat, but you will get a very similar outcome.

CARROT CAKE

created by Kim Campbell in The PlantPure Nation Cookbook

Ingredients:

3 tablespoons flax meal

9 tablespoons (just over ½ cup) hot water

1 cup sucanat

½ cup unsweetened applesauce

1 cup nondairy milk

1 teaspoon vanilla extract

2 cups finely processed or shredded carrots

2 cups whole wheat pastry flour

½ teaspoon sea salt

2 teaspoons baking powder

½ teaspoon baking soda

2 teaspoons pumpkin pie spice

½ cup finely chopped walnuts

½ cup raisins

Directions:

1. Preheat oven to 350 degrees. Line a 9 x 12 pan with parchment paper and set side.

2. In a small bowl, mix together the flax meal and water. Let stand for 1-2 minutes.

3. In a mixing bowl, combine the sucanat, applesauce, milk, vanilla, carrots, and flax meal mixture.

4. In another bowl, combine the flour, salt, baking powder, baking soda, and pumpkin pie spice. Add to the applesauce mixture along with the walnuts and raisins. Gently mix until all the ingredients are wet. Do not overmix.

5. Pour the batter into the prepared pan, smoothing the top with the back of a spoon.

6. Bake for 20-25 minutes, or until a toothpick inserted into the center comes out clean.

CREAMY FROSTING FOR CARROT CAKE

Ingredients:

7 ounces extra-firm tofu

½ cup raw cashews or cashew butter

¼ cup agave nectar

¼ cup water

½ teaspoon vanilla extract

1/8 teaspoon sea salt

Directions:

1. Place all the ingredients into a Vitamix or another high-powered blender and blend until smooth and creamy.

2. Refrigerate for 1-2 hours so the frosting will thicken.

TIPS

This can easily be made into a chocolate frosting by adding ¼ cup or so of unsweetened cocoa powder. How much depends on how dark and rich you want the chocolate flavor.

If you do not have a high-powered blender, you may want to soak the cashews beforehand or use cashew butter instead of raw cashews.

CHOCOLATE PUDDING CAKE

created by Dr. Neal Pinckney from
http://heart.kumu.org/pud.html

This cake reminds me of a lave cake I used to make before I became plant-based.

Ingredients:

1 cup whole wheat pastry flour

2/3 cup sugar

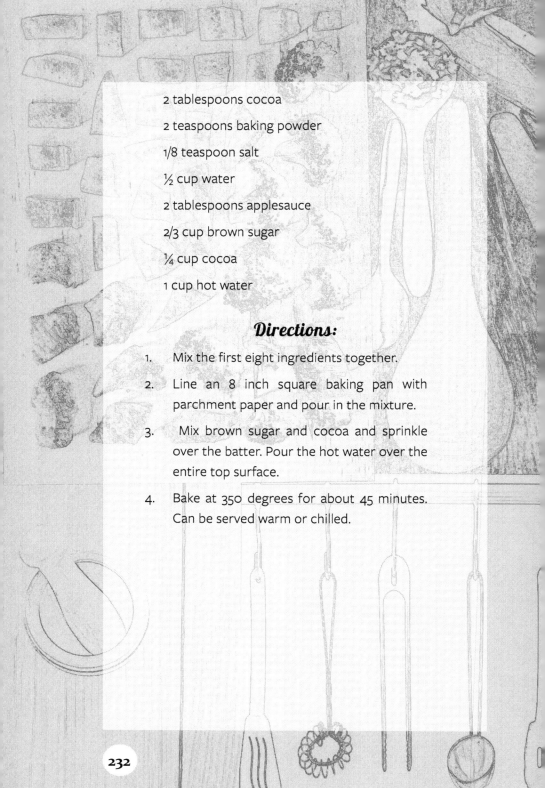

2 tablespoons cocoa

2 teaspoons baking powder

1/8 teaspoon salt

½ cup water

2 tablespoons applesauce

2/3 cup brown sugar

¼ cup cocoa

1 cup hot water

Directions:

1. Mix the first eight ingredients together.

2. Line an 8 inch square baking pan with parchment paper and pour in the mixture.

3. Mix brown sugar and cocoa and sprinkle over the batter. Pour the hot water over the entire top surface.

4. Bake at 350 degrees for about 45 minutes. Can be served warm or chilled.

APPLE CRANBERRY CRISP

creator unknown

Filling:

8 large apples, (mixture of tart and sweet works well), peeled, cored and sliced ½ inch thick

1 cup fresh cranberries

½ - ¾ cup sugar, depending on how sweet apples are that you are using

½ - ¾ cup water (equaling quantity of sugar used above)

2 tablespoons cornstarch or arrow root powder

1 ½ teaspoons cinnamon

1/8 teaspoon nutmeg

1/8 teaspoon cloves

Topping:

1/3 cup almond flour or almond meal

1 cup thinly sliced almonds

1 cup rolled oats

¼ cup pure maple syrup

¼ cup apple sauce

1 teaspoon cinnamon

¼ teaspoon fine grain sea salt

Directions:

1. Preheat oven to 375 degrees.

2. In a large bowl, mix apples, cranberries, cinnamon, nutmeg and cloves.

3. In a small pan, mix sugar, water, and thickener (corn starch or arrow root), cooking until thickened and semi-translucent. When done, spread over the fruit.

4. Mix topping ingredients and crumble over the fruit. If you want a thicker topping layer, you may want to double the topping.

5. Bake 30-40 minutes until filling is bubbling and topping is golden brown. Watch carefully. If the topping is getting too brown, cover with foil for the remainder of the cooking time.

PUMPKIN BUNDT CAKE

created by Erin Hicks Miller and modified by Sherry Shrallow

Ingredients:

½ cup soy or plain almond milk

1 teaspoon nutmeg

1 teaspoon salt

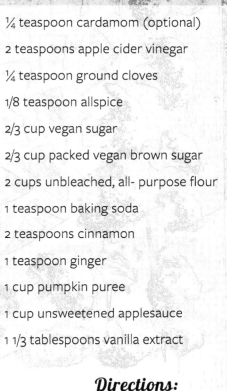

¼ teaspoon cardamom (optional)

2 teaspoons apple cider vinegar

¼ teaspoon ground cloves

1/8 teaspoon allspice

2/3 cup vegan sugar

2/3 cup packed vegan brown sugar

2 cups unbleached, all- purpose flour

1 teaspoon baking soda

2 teaspoons cinnamon

1 teaspoon ginger

1 cup pumpkin puree

1 cup unsweetened applesauce

1 1/3 tablespoons vanilla extract

Directions:

1. Preheat oven to 350 degrees. Use a non-stick bunt pan.

2. In a large measuring cup, combine the soy milk and vinegar to create soy "buttermilk." Set aside to allow to curdle while preparing the rest of the ingredients.

3. In a large mixing bowl, combine the sugars and whisk until smooth. Sift all the additional dry ingredients (including the spices and salt) into the sugars. Whisk to combine.

4. In a small bowl, stir together the pumpkin,

applesauce and vanilla. Pour the wet ingredients into the dry, adding the soy "buttermilk" last. Combine all the ingredients until smooth and pour into bundt cake pan. Bake about 45 minutes. Insert toothpick into thickest part to make sure it is cooked through.

5. Cool for at least one hour before removing cake from pan by inverting and putting on cake plate. It works best to move a knife around the edges of cake while in pan to loosen before inverting. Frost with Maple Glaze below:

Maple Glaze Frosting:

Whisk 1 ½ cups confectioner's sugar with 1/8 cup soy or almond milk and 1 tablespoon maple syrup (Grade B or better). Spoon over cake and spread with back of a spoon or spatula.

SWEET AND SPICY MANGO SORBET

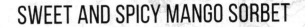

created by *Sherry Shrallow*

Directions:

In a good blender, place the following and blend until smooth. When done, freeze until ready to use.

1 ½ cups frozen mango, slightly thawed

2 ripe bananas (I freeze ripe bananas in small slices and use as needed)

½ cup fresh squeezed lemon juice

¼ - ½ cup agave nectar

Pinch of cayenne pepper

MODIFIED BLACK RUSSIAN CAKE

created by *Dawn Nelson*

Ingredients:

1 yellow Duncan Hines Cake Mix (no pudding)

One 6-ounce Instant chocolate pudding

Ener-G Egg Replacer for four eggs

1 cup apple sauce

½ cup sugar

¼ cup vodka

¼ cup kalua

¾ cup water

Directions:

1. Mix all ingredients for 4 minutes. Pour into bundt pan. Bake at 350 degrees for 55-60 minutes.

2. Beat ¼ cup powdered sugar and ¼ cup kalua in bowl.

3. Cool cake for 15 minutes. Invert and place on serving dish and put 40 fork holes in cake. Drizzle powdered sugar/kalua mix over top and sides of cake. Refrigerate for up to two weeks.

COCONUT MANGO PUDDING

created by LeAnne Campbell from The China Study Cookbook

Ingredients:

¼ cup quick cooking pearl tapioca

¼ teaspoon salt

One 15-ounce can unsweetened coconut milk

(I use light coconut milk)

1 cup fresh or frozen mangos, diced

½ cup sucanat

½ cup soy milk

1 teaspoon vanilla extract

½ teaspoon cinnamon

¼ teaspoon powdered ginger

Fresh mangos and strawberries for topping

Directions:

1. Pour tapioca, salt, coconut milk, mangos and sucanat into saucepan. Boil and then simmer for 12-15 minutes.

2. Add soy milk, vanilla, cinnamon and ginger. Bring back to boil and cook for another 3-5 minutes.

3. Pour into serving dishes and refrigerate until thickened.

4. Garnish with fresh mangos and strawberries if desired.

Endnotes

Chapter 2

1   https://www.heart.org/HEARTORG/Conditions/911-Warnings-Signs-of-a-Heart-Attack_UCM_305346_SubHomePage.jsp

Chapter 4

2   The McDougall Newsletter, Jan 2016, Volume 15, Issue 1: *The Egg Industry: Exposing a Source of Food Poisoning.*

3   http://https://www.hopkinsmedicine.org/heart_vascular_institute/clinical_services/ centers_excellence/ womens_cardiovascular_health_center/patient_information/health_topics/depression_heart_ disease.html

4   https://www.heart.org/HEARTORG/HealthyLiving/StressManagement/HowDoesStressAffectYou/Depression-After-A-Cardiac-Event-or-Diagnosis_UCM_440444_Article.jsp#.WWt-hYWcGUk

Chapter 6

5   Esselstyn, Jr, Caldwell, MD, "Prevent and Reverse Heart Disease, The Revolutionary, Scientifically Proven, Nutrition-based Cure," Published by the Penguin Group, 2007.

6   Esselstyn CB Jr. "Updating a 12 – Year Experience With Arrest and Reversal Therapy for Coronary Heart Disease (An Overdue Requiem for palliative Cardiology)" *The American Journal of Cardiology*, 1999 August 1; 84:339-41.

7   Esselstyn CB Jr. "A Way to Prevent CAD?," *The Journal of Family Practice.* July 2014 Vol 63. No 7 page 257

8   Dean Ornish, MD; Larry W. Scherwitz, PhD; James H. Billings, PhD, MPH; et al "Intensive Lifestyle Changes for Reversal of Coronary Heart Disease" *JAMA*, 1998;280(23):2001-2007. doi:10.1001/jama280.23.2001.

9   https://www.medicalnewsinc.com/clinical/article/20489454/healthways-expands-dr-dean-ornishs-program-for-reversing-heart-disease-for-cardiac-patients

10   https://hpjmh.com/2013/05/20/plant-based-for-all-patients-says-kaiser-permanente/

11   https://my.clevelandclinic.org/departments/wellness/integrative/disease-reversal

12   https://www.health.harvard.edu/heart-health/halt-heart-disease-with-a-

plant-based-oil-free-diet-

13   https://www.pcrm.org/media/news/ama-passes-resolution-hospitals-
         should-provide-plant-based-meals-and-remove-cancer-causing-processed

14   *See* Esselstyn, *supra.*

15   https://www.ornish.com/zine/new-scientifically-validated-guidelines-
         nuts-and-seeds/

16   *See* Esselstyn, *supra.*

17   https://www.drcarney.com/blog/entry/the-effect-of-different-oils-on-
         endothelial-function

18   https://nutritionstudies.org/provocations-casein-carcinogen-really/

19   https://www.pcrm.org/health/diets/vegdiets/how-can-i-get-enough-
         protein-the-protein-myth

20   Campbell, T. Colin, Ph.D., Campbell, Thomas M. II, *The China Study: The
         Most Comprehensive Study of Nutrition Ever Conducted and the Starling
         Implications for Diet, Weight Loss and Long-term Health,"* published by
         BenBella Books, Inc. 2006

21   *See* Esselstyn, *supra.*

22   *See* Esselstyn, *supra.*

Chapter 9

23   https://www.pcrm.org/media/news/physicians-committee-sues-usda-
         and-dhhs

24   https://www.cnpp.usda.gov/2015-2020-dietary-guidelines-americans

25   https://time.com/4130043/lobbying-politics-dietary-guidelines/

26   https://circ.ahajournals.org/content/circulationaha/99/6/779.full.pdf

27   https://www.heart.org/HEARTORG/General/About-Us---American-
         Heart-Association_UCM_305422_SubHomePage.jsp

28   Ramon Estruch, M.D., Pph.D., Emilio Ros, M.D., Ph.D., Jordi Salas-Salvado,
         M.D., Ph.D., Maria-Isabel Covas, D.Pharm., Ph.D., Dodlores Corella, D.
         Pharm., Ph.D., Fernando Aros, M.D., Ph.D., Enrique Gomez-Garcia, M.D.,
         Ph.D., Valentina Ruiz Gut-Gutierrez, Ph.D., Miquel Fiol., M.D., Ph.D., Jose
         Lapetra., M.D., Ph.D., Rosa Maria Lamuela-Raventos, D.Phar,., Ph.D., Lluis
         Serra-Mejam, M.D., Ph.D., Xavier Pinto, M.D., Ph.D., Joseph Basaro, M.D.,
         Ph.D., Miguel Angel Munoz, M.D., Ph.D., Jose V. Sorli, M.D., Ph.D., Jose
         Alfredo Martinez, M.D., Ph.D., and Miguel Angell Martinez-Gonzalez,
         M.D., Ph.D. et al., for the PREDIMED Study Investigators "Primary
         Prevention of Cardiovascular Disease with a Mediterranean Diet," *The New
         England Journal of Medicine*, 2013; 368:1279-1290.

29   Kim T.B. Knoops, MSc; Lisette C.P.G.M. de Groot, Ph.D: Daan
        Kromhout, PhD; Anne-Elisabeth Perrin, MD, MSc; Olga Moreiras-
        Varela, PhD; Alessandro Menotti, MD, PHD; Wija A. van Staveren, PhD.
        "Mediterranean Diet, Lifestyle Factors, and 10-Year Mortality in Elderly
        European men and Women: The HALE project" JAMA, 2004; 292(12):
        1433-1439.

30   American Heart Association and Jennie Garth, "American Heart
        Association The Go Red For Women Cookbook: Cooking Your Way to a
        Heart-Healthy Weight and Good Nutrition," 2013

Chapter 10

31   Bussone, Danielle, *Time For Change*, published by DanRick Publishing, 2015.

32   https://www.pbs.org/wnet/need-to-know/health/the-dirty-dozen-and-
        clean-15-of-produce/616/

Chapter 12

33   https://nutritionstudies.org/12-frightening-facts-milk/

34   https://www.insidermonkey.com/blog/11-countries-with-the-highest-
        rates-of-osteoporosis-in-the-world-359037/11/

35   https://www.riseofthevegan.com

Chapter 13

36   McDougall, John, "Vitamin D Supplements are Harmful: Sunshine
        and Food Determine Health," *McDougall's Health and Medical Center
        Newsletter*, March 31, 2015.

37   Montgomery, Baxter, D., *The Food Prescription for Better Health*,
        published by Delworth Publishing, 2001 pp. 142

Chapter 14

38   "Breathing-Based Meditation Decreases Posttraumatic Stress Disorder
        Symptoms in U.S. Military Veterans: A Randomized Controlled
        Longitudinal Study," Emma M Seppälä, Jack B Nitschke, Dana L
        Tudorascu, Andrea Hayes, Michael R Goldstein, Dong T H Nguyen,
        David Perlman, and Richard J Davidson Journal of Traumatic Stress, 2014
        August; 27(4); 397-405

Chapter 17

39   *See* Esselstyn *supra*.
40   *See* Campbell, *supra*, pp.99-101.

RESOURCES

The China Study: The Most Comprehensive Study of Nutrition Ever Conducted And the Startling Implications for Diet by T. Colin Campbell, Thomas M. Campbell II, Howard Lyman and John Robbins (May 11, 2006).

Prevent and Reverse Heart Disease: The Revolutionary Scientifically Proven, Nutrition-Based Cure by Caldwell Esselstyn Jr. M.D. (February 1, 2007).

The McDougall Plan by John A. McDougall and Mary A. McDougall (October 22, 1983).

The Starch Solution: Eat The Foods You Love, Regain Your Health, and Lose the Weight for Good! by John McDougall and Mary McDougall (May 8, 2012).

Dr. Dean Ornish's Program For Reversing Heart Disease by Dr. Dean Ornish (September 22, 2010).

Time For Change by Danielle Bussone (2015).

The Food Prescription for Better Health: A Cardiologist's Proven Method to Reverse Heart Disease, Diabetes, Obesity, and Other Chronic Illnesses, Naturally! by Baxter D. Montgomery, MD (2011).

How Not To Die by Michael Greger, M.D. with Gene Stone (2015).

The Campbell Plan by Thomas Campbell, MD (2015).

The Pleasure Trap- Mastering the Hidden Force That Undermines Health & Happiness by Douglas J. Lisle Ph.D. and Alan Goldhamer DC (2003).

Unprocessed: How to achieve vibrant health and your ideal weight by Chef A.J. and Glen Merzer (2011).

Dr. Neal Barnard's Program for Reversing Diabetes: The Scientifically Proven System for Reversing Diabetes without Drugs by Dr. Neal Barnard (2008).

Power Foods For The Brain: An Effective 3-Step Plan to Protect Yur Mind and Strengthen Your Memory by Dr. Neal Barnard (2014).

The Cheese Trap: How Breaking a Surprising Addiction Will Help You Lose Weight, Gain Energy and Strengthen Your Memory, by Dr. Neal Barnard (2014).

COOKBOOKS USING NO OIL

Prevent and Reverse Heart Disease: The Revolutionary Scientifically Proven, Nutrition-Based Cure by Caldwell Esselstyn Jr. M.D. (February 1, 2007).

The Prevent and Reverse Heart Disease Cookbook by Ann Crile Esselstyn and Jane Esselstyn (2014).

Forks Over Knives The Cookbook by Del Sroufe with Desserts by Isa Chandra Moskowitz (2012).

The China Study Cookbook by LeAnne Campbell, PhD (2013).

The China Study Family Cookbook by Del Sroufe (2017).

The China Study Quick and Easy Cookbook by Del Sroufe (2015).

The PlantPure Nation Cookbook by Kim Campbell (2015).

The McDougall Quick and Easy Cookbook by John A. McDougall and Mary McDougall (1997).

The New McDougall Cookbook by John A. McDougall and Mary McDougall (1993).

Straight Up Food: Delicious and Easy Plant-based Cooking without Salt, Oil or Sugar by Cathy Fisher (2016).

The Engine 2 Cookbook by Rip Esselstyn and Jane Esselstyn (2017).

How Not To Die Cookbook by Dr. Michael Greger (2017).

WEBSITES

https://www.fatfreevegan.com
https://www.vegfamily.com
https://www.wholefoods.com/recipes
https://www.chooseveg.com
https://www.midwestveg.com
https://simple-veganista.com
https://www.runningonrealfood.com
https://www.engine2.com
https://lifestylemedicine.org
http://vegdocs.com/
https://www.wellnessforum.com
https://www.drmcdougall.com
https://www.pcrm.org
https://www.nutritionfacts.org
https://www.thevegan8.com
https://www.vegginoutandabout.com
https://www.timeforchangekitchen.com
https://happyherbivore.com/recipes
https://www.brandnewvegan.com/recipe-index
https://www.feastingonfruit.com/recipe-index/
https://www.straightupfood.com/blog/recipe-index/
https://dreenaburton.com/plant-powered-kitchen/
https://www.cearaskitchen.com/category/all-recipes/
https://cookingwithplants.com/
https://myplantbasedfamily.com/
https://www.nutriplanet.org/
https://theplantphilosophy.com/
https://sharan-india.org/
https://nutritionstudies.org/
https://sandysveganblogsandblahs.blogspot.com/
https://www.rawtillwhenever.com/
https://www.fullyraw.com/recipes-list/

https://riseshinecook.ca/blog/
https://www.plants-rule.com/
https://sweetsimplevegan.com/
https://plantbasedcookingshow.com/
https://potatostrong.com/plant-based-low-fat-oil-recipes/
https://eatplant-based.com/
https://www.veggieinspired.com/
https://www.22daysnutrition.com/
https://engine2diet.com/blog/category/recipes/
https://simpledailyrecipes.com/
https://www.plantplate.com/
https://healthygirlskitchen.com/healthy-recipes
https://helynskitchen.com/
https://nutmegnotebook.com/
https://jewishfoodhero.com/
https://whitneyross@mac.com/
https://oneingredientchef.com/
https://www.happyhealthylonglife.com/about.html
https://myvegancookbook.com/
https://heart.kumu.org/
https://www.jeffnovick.com
https://www.happycow.net
https://www.sageplantpoweredhealth.com
https://vegjauntsandjourneys.com/

WELLNESS RETREATS

https://www.taosyogaretreat.com Taos Yoga Retreat is a residential private retreat center in Taos, New Mexico led by Ceily Levy. It offers yoga, meditation and complimentary practices. For those seeking the wisdom of an awakened life it is a haven for the path of a compassionate living practice, the healing presence of nature and the study of techniques that cultivate wellbeing and resilience. Welcoming experienced and beginning practitioners.

Qi Gong is an ancient practice of health, energy and vitality from China that strengthens your body, mind and emotions. April Day Epstein, a former dancer, has trained and become certified to teach Qi Gong from Master Lee Holden. April's 35 years of teaching movement to students of all ages and levels speaks to her life's passion for helping others connect to their inner sense of self and wisdom. For more information please contact April at aprilepstein@sbcglobal.net.

DOCUMENTARIES

Forks Over Knives
Food Inc.
Fast Food Nation,
Fat Sick and Nearly Dead
Vegucated
Cowspiracy
PlantPure Nation
What The Health
Food Matters
Simply Raw: Reversing Diabetes in 30 Days
Ingredients
The Future of Food
Hungry for Change
Earthlings
The Engine2 Kitchen Rescue
The Game Changers
Eating You Alive

54431261R00146